Never Give Up

"We know without question that cancer patients with a strong will to recover do better than patients who don't care or think it's all up to their doctors. A courageous attitude and a willingness to follow a prescribed course of medical therapy yields more positive results than any other form of treatment.

"Your battle against cancer is one you probably never thought you'd have to undertake. Marshal all your reserves—your intelligence, your basic health, your spirit and drive—and give this battle everything you've got.

"Whatever your prognosis, remember that the key word is 'hope.' NEVER GIVE UP. More women than ever before are living happy, productive lives for many years after their breast cancer was initially diagnosed.

"Good luck to you."

—Dr. Carol Fabian

Other books in the *Recovering From* series:

Recovering From A Stroke
*Recovering From Coronary Bypass Surgery
*Recovering From A Hysterectomy

Published by
HarperPaperbacks

*coming soon

RECOVERING FROM BREAST CANCER

CAROL FABIAN, M.D.
ANDREA WARREN, M.A., M.S.

HarperPaperbacks
A Division of HarperCollinsPublishers

HarperPaperbacks   *A Division of* HarperCollins*Publishers*
                     10 East 53rd Street, New York, N.Y. 10022

Cover design by Richard Rossiter

First printing: March 1992

Printed in the United States of America

HarperPaperbacks and colophon are trademarks of
HarperCollins*Publishers*

10 9 8 7 6 5 4 3 2 1

To all of the women who have bravely battled or are battling the disease of breast cancer, and to all of the members of the medical community who are working tirelessly in a unified quest to eradicate it, thank you for your inspiration.

ACKNOWLEDGMENTS

The authors would like to thank the following people for their assistance and support in the writing of this book:

Eileen Fallon
Janice Foster
Lester Garfinkle, M.D.
Barbara Gill, RN., M.S.N.
Amy Strauss Tranin, RN., M.S., O.C.N.

And a very special thanks to Kim Fulk.

CONTENTS

CONTENTS

INTRODUCTION

You are probably reading this book because you or a loved one have been recently diagnosed with breast cancer. The more you know about the disease, your allies in the medical community, and about your own mind and body, the more chance of full recovery you have.

Our knowledge about breast cancer increases every day. Even as you read this, new technology is being perfected to assist in diagnosis and treatment. But medical science can take you only so far. The rest is up to you.

More women than ever are surviving breast cancer and living happy, productive lives. A positive outlook and close involvement in your own treatment combined with first-rate medical care give you the best chance of recovery.

We believe that the recovery process should begin with diagnosis. We're going to explore with you (or a friend or loved one who may be reading this book) what's happening to your body, what treatment options modern medicine offers you, and how your psychological health affects your ability to combat this disease.

—Carol Fabian, M.D., and Andrea Warren

! Physical Recovery

1 How You Got Breast Cancer

No woman forgets the moment when she hears the news that she has breast cancer. It doesn't matter who's with her at the time or where she is, the overwhelming impact of the words often makes it impossible for her to hear anything else that is said to her.

Invariably, one of her first thoughts is, "Am I going to die?" And even if she's reassured that her chances of survival are very very good—indeed, overwhelmingly good—doubt often creeps in.

You know, because it's happened to you. Only people who have been told they have cancer can understand how terrifying this experience is.

Cancer, after all, is a very scary word. At one time it meant almost certain death, because doctors had limited means to treat it. We've all known or heard of someone who got cancer and died from it once cancer spread throughout the person's body. Sometimes this happened over the course of years and sometimes it happened very rapidly.

Most of us also know at least one exception—someone who had cancer and lived with it trouble-free until the end of a long, fairly healthy life.

Recovery Begins with Diagnosis

Wherever you are in your battle against breast cancer, and whatever your prognosis, chances are the first thing you thought when you received this news was that you were going to die.

As you recovered a little from your shock, and as you've learned more about breast cancer, you've found out that many women successfully conquer this disease. The war you must wage against this disease is both physical and psychological. The more you know about breast cancer and about what's happening to your body, the more you can participate in your treatment and interact positively with your medical team.

Knowledge is power!

A Disease As Old As Humankind

As far as we know, cancer has always been present in humans. Scientists have found evidence of cancer in Egyptian mummies over five thousand years old. They've even found it in dinosaur bones.

We don't know when breast cancer was first diagnosed. Before the development of anesthesia, surgical methods were primitive, and most women probably eventually died of their disease rather than endure breast amputation.

In the late 1890s, a surgeon named William Halsted utilized the development of anesthesia to perfect the Halsted mastectomy method still in use today. Unfortunately, many women with breast cancer denied themselves treatment because for a long time it was considered a venereal disease.

Although women today do not consider breast cancer a venereal disease, many are still uneasy about someone other than their husbands, lovers, or themselves touching their breasts. This complicates efforts by health educators to teach women how to do breast self-exams and to go to their physicians for yearly breast exams.

In spite of its long history, cancer is still cloaked in mystery, myths, and misconceptions. While we are learning more about it all the time, there is still much we don't know about both its causes and its treatment.

A Hundred Diseases

Even the term "cancer" is misleading, for it's actually over a hundred different diseases. Each may have a different natural history and respond differently to treatment. There are several types of breast cancer as well. The common characteristic that links and defines cancer is the abnormal growth of cells that invade and destroy healthy body tissue.

Some cancer cells grow slowly, while others grow very quickly. Often their growth rate varies over time, going from slow to fast and back again, or vice versa. Cancer cells are out of control. They don't grow the way

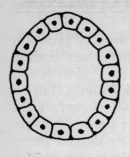

Normal duct

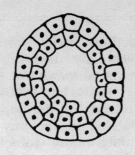

Hyperplastic duct

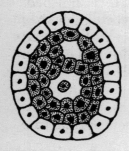

Carcinoma in situ

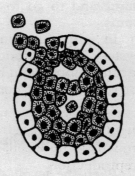

Invasive breast cancer

illustration 1: Round to square-shaped cells line the breast ducts. Normal duct: In a normal duct, the cells are fairly uniform in size and shape. Hyperplastic duct: When the cells begin to grow, the individual cells look normal but begin to pile up in the duct.

Cancer cells are abnormal in shape and size and don't stick well together. Carcinoma in situ: Cancer cells are contained within the duct wall lining. Invasive breast cancer: Cancer cells invade outside the duct wall.

they're supposed to, nor do they stop growing when they should. They begin to compete with healthy cells for space and nutrients. Eventually, as tumors form, they destroy the healthy cells. (See Illustration #1.)

How Healthy Cells Work

Normal body cells work constantly to replace worn-out cells in the body, maintaining a balance between the old and the new. Healthy cells have what can most easily be explained as receptors that receive and obey signals from other organs and tissue cells in the body.

Some kinds of cells can actually regenerate if the body is injured and cells are destroyed. Other types of cells stop growing once the body's growth is finished. Still others can increase the rapidity with which they reproduce when the body needs them. For example, red blood cells, which carry oxygen, can reproduce seven times faster than normal in response to bleeding. White cells also reproduce rapidly when they have an infection to fight. When the stress is over, the tissue or organs from which these cells arose return to their normal rate of reproduction.

If normal cells are surrounded by cancer cells, the normal cells may not be able to perform their work. We think that cancer cells may secrete substances that can cause healthy cells to break down. Then the cancer cells can invade the healthy tissue.

Cancer confined to the breast is not fatal. But if the cancer cells move to any of the vital organs, such as the brain, liver, lungs, or bone marrow, the body begins to lose its ability to function normally. It is the destruction of these vital life processes that makes cancer a killer.

But Why Does a Cell Become Cancerous?

Why does a normal cell malfunction and become cancerous? Why do some people with long-term exposure to known cancer-causing agents, such as cigarettes or the sun, get cancer, while others do not?

We don't know exactly, but it seems to be related to a person's ability to repair mutations or accidents these substances cause in the cells of the body. It may also be that some people's bodies can somehow control the cell growth that can lead to cancer.

The presence of all of the following items may be necessary before a person will develop a cancer in their body that has the potential to spread to other body organs:

1. An accident or mutation in the normal cells' genetic material, which is called DNA.
2. The inability of the cell to repair itself after the accident.
3. The inability of the cells to respond to normal negative controls on growth.
4. The inability of the body's immune system to destroy the abnormal cells.
5. The ability of these abnormal cells to secrete substances, called proteases, which break down normal body tissues and allow these cells to get out into the bloodstream where they can travel to distant organ sites.

Even though these "abnormal" or potentially cancerous cells arise thousands of times in a person's lifetime, it is fortunately a very rare event when all five conditions are operative at once.

Most of these genetic accidents that lead to cancer happen in the genes that normally switch growth on and off at periodic intervals during a person's lifetime. It usually takes a combination of several "accidents" in the "switch on" genes (oncogenes) combined with loss or accidents in the "switch off" genes (tumor suppressor or anti-oncogenes), combined with conditions two to five, to produce cancer.

Initiators and Promoters

Substances that make the genetic material susceptible to breaks or accidents can help *initiate* cancer. Examples of such initiators are some viruses, radiation, some types of chemotherapy, and other types of chemicals, such as those found in cigarettes.

Other substances simply cause growth when there normally would be little or no growth, or cause faster growth than normal. Estrogen in postmenopausal women and too much fat in the diet and body may be examples. Such a substance is called a *promoter*. Because more cells are growing faster than normal, the chances are greater that *initiators* can work on the genetic material.

Sometimes a person's own heredity works against him or her. Cancer can definitely "run in families." Most cancers, however, are spontaneous. Families that tend to have a large amount of cancer may have inheritable defects in an "off switch" gene (tumor suppressor) which, combined with promoter and/or initiator substances, leads to cancer.

It only takes one cancer cell to start the tumor

growth. That cell multiplies into two cells. They multiply into four cells, and so forth. Not all the cells grow and divide at any one time. It may be that as few as 2 percent or as many as 50 percent are active at a given time. It can take anywhere from two years to twenty years for a cancerous lump in the breast to reach the size where it can be felt with the fingertips.

Ongoing research will hopefully provide specific answers in the near future that may help medical science stop cancer before it ever starts.

Benign Versus Malignant

When referring to the breasts, the term "lump" means something we can feel. It may be a solid mass, called a tumor, or a cyst.

A cyst is filled with liquid or semisolid material. About 30 percent of all women develop breast cysts at one time or another. Some women get them repeatedly. Only rarely do they become cancerous. However, women prone to getting them run a slightly higher risk than average of developing breast cancer sometime in their lives.

A tumor is made up of cells. Most tumors are *benign*, which means they are not cancerous. Sometimes they cause no problems at all. But if they grow in a contained space, like the brain, or if they press on vital organs, they can be dangerous and must be surgically removed. If they are removed, usually they do not return.

A primary difference between benign and malignant (cancerous) tumors is that malignant tumors have the ability to spread to other organs. The organ in which the first cancerous tumor forms in the body is referred to as the *primary* site of the cancer, and where it grows is referred to as a tumor bed. Any other tumors that grow elsewhere in the body as a result of cancerous cells breaking away from the primary tumor will have the parent tumor's characteristics.

This means that if you have breast cancer and it spreads to the lungs, your tumor in the lung will be referred to as breast cancer metastatic to the lung, not as lung cancer. The lung tumors will respond to similar chemicals as does the original breast cancer.

How Cancer Spreads

If you have heard of someone dying from breast cancer, it may be confusing to realize that breast cancer itself doesn't kill. Rather, the breast cancer *metastasizes*, or spreads, beyond the breast or breasts to one or more vital organs. The cancer then destroys that vital organ or those organs, and we cannot live without it or them.

Breast cancer spreads to these organs in one of two ways:

1. The cancer cells grow by direct extension, invading a vital organ.
2. Cancerous cells from the primary tumor invade the lymph nodes or the blood vessels, and from there travel to other parts of the body where they may form more tumors.

Not many of the cancerous cells that undertake this journey through the lymph system or the bloodstream survive, because the body's immune system mounts its defenses to fight them. But if a few make it and become lodged somewhere, they may begin to multiply again—even though they're far away from the primary tumor—

11

and form new malignant tumors that begin attacking the healthy tissues around them.

It's the cancer cells that enter the blood vessels that pose the greatest risk, because the bloodstream can carry them to every organ in the body.

Breast Cancer in American Women

Cancer can occur almost anywhere in the body. It occurs in the breasts with alarming frequency. According to statistics, one in every ten women in the United States will develop breast cancer and it accounts for one-fourth of all cancers in women.

Every year, doctors diagnose approximately 150,000 cases of breast cancer in American women. Without treatment of any kind, about 95 percent of these women would eventually die from the disease. With early detection and treatment, a minimum of 80 percent of women can be cured of the disease.

Where in the Breast Does Cancer Develop?

The breast is composed of a system of lobules—little bulblike structures that can produce milk. The lobules are connected by ducts to the nipple, making it possible for a baby to nurse. Fat fills in the spaces between the ducts in the breast. (See Illustration #2.)

Ninety percent of all breast cancers develop in the lining of the ducts or lobules and are referred to as ductal cancer or lobular cancer, respectively.

The first signs of breast cancer may be a change in the size or shape of the breast or a change in color or

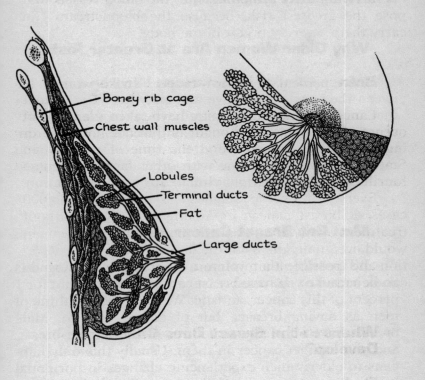

Boney rib cage

Chest wall muscles

Lobules

Terminal ducts

Fat

Large ducts

illustration 2: As a cross section of a mature female breast shows, the breast is composed of a system of ducts and lobules that allow a woman to manufacture milk and nurse a baby. Fat and connective tissue fill in the rest of the breast space. Breast cancer most often arises in the part of the terminal duct next to the lobule.

texture of the skin or nipple, a lump or thickening in the breast or armpit, or nipple discharge. Pain in the breast is rarely an early symptom.

Why Older Women Are at Greater Risk

Fifty percent of breast cancers strike women between the ages of forty-five and sixty-five. The changes that initiated the cancer may have taken place twenty years earlier. Current thought is that the hormone imbalances that occur around the time of puberty and menopause may combine with other factors discussed earlier to create the right climate for cancer initiation.

Men Get Breast Cancer, Too

It's possible that you're a man who's reading this book because you have breast cancer. Men account for 1 percent of this cancer statistic. We don't usually think of men as having breasts, but of course you do. Male breasts have all of the structures of the female breast, and you can get cancer in them. Usually this only happens to elderly men experiencing changes in hormonal levels. Present in men's testes are cells producing estrogen as well as cells producing testosterone. As men age, the cells producing testosterone (the male hormone) often atrophy and cease testosterone production before cells producing estrogen. This hormonal imbalance in the testicles may be an important promotional factor that causes breast cancer in men.

Because you make up so small a minority of breast cancer patients, we will continue to refer to readers of this book as women. But be assured that we know you're out there, and that much of what we have to say relates to you, too.

Other Contributing Factors

As discussed earlier in this chapter, a large number of factors may have provided the right climate for you to develop breast cancer.

If you have a family history of breast cancer, perhaps you inherited genetic material with malfunctions in one or more tumor suppressor genes. Or accidents or mutations in the tumor suppressor genes may simply have occurred spontaneously sometime in your lifetime.

You may have ingested cancer-causing substances or eaten a high fat diet that made your breast growth genes work overtime. Perhaps your natural body chemistry provided you with an estrogen-progesterone imbalance. In any event, the larger the proportion of breast cells that are growing, the greater the chance that permanent genetic alterations will occur during cell division.

The role of certain viral infections in breast cancer is not as clear as for some other cancers. Certain viruses can permanently insert themselves into a person's genetic material. When they do, they can cause the oncogenes to switch into their "growth on" state permanently and uncontrollably. Or they can bind to and tie up the protein messengers of the tumor suppressor "growth off" genes so that they cannot do their work.

Categories That Put You at Risk

About 25 percent of women who develop breast cancer have an identifiable major risk factor, and 75 percent do not. In spite of what we don't yet know about breast cancer, we do know that the major risk factors for women include previous breast cancer and/or a family history of cancer. Women who have been diagnosed as having atypical hyperplasia on a breast biopsy are also at increased risk.

Family history is especially important if a woman's mother or sister has or had breast cancer. This risk is especially significant if the cancer occurred in both breasts and/or the mother or sister had not yet gone through menopause.

Once a woman has cancer in one breast, she stands at least a 13 percent chance of developing it in the other one. If in addition she has a mother or sister with breast cancer, the risk of a new cancer in the remaining breast may go to 20 percent or higher.

Minor factors that put a woman at slightly higher than normal risk include:

- A high fat diet, especially if the woman is overweight.
- Obesity.
- Smoking.
- Alcohol.
- Early menstruation (age eleven or earlier) or late menopause.
- Childlessness or giving birth to a first child after age thirty.
- Estrogen replacement in postmenopausal women

may also be associated with a higher-than-normal risk.

Some of these "minor" factors can be controlled by life-style choices. Because they may be "tumor promoters," they may assume particular importance in a woman who has one or more major factors already present.

What DIDN'T Give You Breast Cancer

It's time to lay to rest the notion that we somehow wish cancer upon ourselves. Cancer happens because of erratic cell formation. *You didn't make it happen because of your thoughts.*

Nor is cancer caused by injury to the breasts. Bumping, bruising, or cuts may hurt you, but they heal and they do *not* cause cancer. Nor does touching the breasts, childbirth, nursing, or having sexual relations cause cancer.

And cancer is *not* contagious. No one can catch it from someone else. Although the predisposition to cancer may be inherited, you will not necessarily pass it on to any daughters you may have.

In spite of concern that radiation involved in mammography might increase the risk of breast cancer, extensive studies show that the benefits from early detection far outweigh the risks of cancer induction. An estimated six cancers are induced per one million screenings. Depending on the age group, 350 to 1,200 cancers will be detected in one million screenings.

Remember: You have no reason to feel guilty or ashamed about having breast cancer. The important thing is that you know you have it and are undergoing treatment so that you can recover from it.

Questions to Ask Your Doctor

At the end of each chapter you'll see suggested questions you may want to ask your doctor. But right now, since the remaining material in the book may answer your questions, we suggest you begin by evaluating your own health history. The more you know about this, and your family's cancer history, the more you'll be able to assist your doctor in determining the best course of treatment for you.

Reviewing your history may also help you eliminate factors that did not influence your getting breast cancer, thus putting your mind at rest.

If you're unsure of your family's health history, you may want to contact a relative who knows more. What you especially want to know is whether there is breast cancer in your family. If so, how old was the relative when she got it? Did the tumor involve one or both breasts?

You may also want to check with a former doctor if you think you have been given supplemental estrogen but aren't sure or if you have previously had your ovaries removed. Also, if you have had a prior biopsy or mammogram, get those reports for your doctor.

With this clear picture of your past, you can help your doctor so that together you can work toward your recovery.

2 Communicating with Health Professionals

As a cancer patient, you're going to hear lots of medical terms that you need to understand in order to communicate with the doctors, nurses, and medical personnel who will be caring for you.

Understanding the Terms

While all of these people should always talk to you in language you clearly understand, you'll probably still hear terms you don't know. In the beginning, ask for an explanation when you hear a word you don't know. Don't be shy about this. It's very important that you clearly communicate with each health-care professional involved in your care, and sometimes they get rushed, or they simply forget that they're using terms foreign to you.

To understand breast cancer diagnosis and treatment in depth, it's helpful first to develop a general understanding about these subjects. They will be covered in depth in later chapters.

Diagnosis

Once a suspicious mass is found in one of your breasts either by exam or mammogram, your doctor must determine if it is cancerous. Fluid-filled cysts are usually not cancerous. But a solid mass can be benign or cancerous.

Often the first procedure done to determine whether a mass is malignant (cancerous) or not is a *needle aspiration*. This is done in the doctor's office with the doctor using a long thin needle with a syringe on the end to attempt to withdraw fluid or cells (the aspirate) from the mass.

The aspirate is then examined under a microscope to see if there are any malignant cells in it. If there are, the next step is usually a *biopsy*.

A biopsy removes the abnormal tissue that was felt by exam or seen on a mammogram. You may wonder why a biopsy is necessary if the aspirate already shows malignant cells. There are several reasons:

1. To determine if the cancer is invasive (i.e., can potentially invade other body organs).
2. To help tell doctors how your cancer is likely to behave.

3. To remove the cancer, but allow you time to decide what type of breast operation to have.

Sometimes doctors bypass aspiration and go directly to biopsy. The biopsy may be done under local or general anesthetic, depending on the size and location of the mass and on patient preference.

If laboratory evaluation shows the mass to be a cancerous tumor, *hormone receptor tests* will be run on it to determine if proteins that are called *receptors* are present. If they are, these receptors will give doctors valuable information because they combine with the female hormones estrogen and progesterone. We know that tumors that are *hormone receptor positive* may grow faster when exposed to estrogen. If the tumor is hormone receptor positive (and tests will determine this), exposing the tumor to drugs called anti-estrogens may suppress growth of the tumor and therefore be part of your treatment.

These tests, along with some other tests that indirectly measure the growth rate (by a strange-sounding procedure called *flow cytometry*) will also help predict your chances of early recurrence of your cancer.

The pathologist, who is a doctor with special training in diagnosing diseased tissue, helps your doctor determine the extent, or *stage*, of the cancer. These stages can range from *carcinoma in situ*, the earliest, most easily cured cancer, to *Stage IV* cancer, which means the cancer has spread to other organs in the body. The stages are discussed in detail in Chapter Three.

Surgical Options

Armed with this basic information, you and your doctor will decide what kind of treatment to begin. Usually the choice is surgery. Your options include the following:

Radical Mastectomy: Removal of the entire breast and nipple, two chest wall muscles, and the lymph nodes under the arm.

Modified Radical Mastectomy: Removal of the entire breast and nipple, one chest wall muscle, and the lymph nodes under the arm.

Simple or Total Mastectomy: Removal of the entire breast and nipple. Usually the lymph nodes under the arm are also removed. If they are, the procedure is called an *extended simple mastectomy.*

Lumpectomy: Also called *partial mastectomy.* Removal of the lump while preserving most of the breast. Lumpectomies are usually combined with *axillary dissection.* This refers to the removal of lymph nodes under the arm.

Breast Reconstruction

If the decision is to perform a mastectomy, you will want to decide whether to begin the process of *breast reconstruction* at the time of your mastectomy or wait until all needed treatment including chemotherapy is completed.

Breast reconstruction is the creation of a mound on the chest wall to simulate the breast—a process that has improved immensely in the past few years.

Adjuvant Therapy

Follow-up treatment, referred to as adjuvant therapy, for your cancer may include one or more of the following:

Radiation Therapy: External treatment with high-energy X rays (radiation) to destroy cancer cells. In addition to radiation by machine, some women receive *interstitial implants* that are surgically inserted into the breast at the actual site (or tumor bed) where the cancerous lump originated.

The purpose of the implant is to deliver a very large dose of radiation to the area most likely to be contaminated with cancer cells.

Chemotherapy: A program of treatment with anticancer drugs usually administered either by mouth or by injection into a vein.

Hormone Therapy: Removing or adding hormones or antihormones to your course of treatment.

Physical Therapy: A program to help you regain full physical use of one or both arms if they were weakened by surgery.

That, in briefest terms, is what happens during cancer treatment. When you finish treatment, your doctor will continue to follow you closely for any signs that cancer might be recurring locally or at a distant site. You will need at least a yearly evaluation of your remaining normal breast for life to make sure a new cancer does not develop.

Your Medical Team

While you are being treated for breast cancer, you will get to know many members of the medical team, including a variety of doctors, nurses, technicians, and office staff. All of these people will be important to you. One doctor, however, needs to be in charge. Who that is depends on where you are in your diagnosis and treatment.

At the hub, initially, will be your *primary-care physician*. This might be a general practice doctor, internist, or surgeon.

Oncologists: Cancer Specialists

After diagnosis and possibly before definitive surgery, you and your doctor will probably decide that you should consult an *oncologist*. This is a physician with a specialty in cancer treatment. There are three types: medical, surgical, and radiation. They usually work closely together.

The medical oncologist is an internist who subspecializes in cancer treatment. He or she is usually responsible for administering hormone or chemotherapy if needed.

The surgical oncologist is a surgeon who confines his practice to the treatment and surgical removal of tumors.

A radiation oncologist delivers the radiation to the cancer or tissue around the original cancer.

Even if your doctor doesn't recommend that you see an oncologist, you should consider doing so anyway. It doesn't mean you don't trust your doctor. It merely means that you recognize what a complicated disease cancer is, and in order to get the best possible treatment, you would like to be in the care of a specialist whose expertise is cancer.

You may want to consult with a *surgical oncologist* who specializes in breast cancer surgery. If lumpectomy is an option for you, you will also see a *radiation oncologist* who will plan your radiation treatment. If you are contemplating mastectomy with breast reconstruction, you may also see a *plastic surgeon*. You may see a medical oncologist after the biopsy even before the definitive surgery to discuss possible treatment after surgery and what effect this might have on the surgical procedure you choose.

Your Medical Team

Ideally, then, you will work with a team of physicians. Your family doctor or your medical or surgical oncologist eventually will oversee and coordinate your entire treatment plan.

When one of these oncologists directs and coordinates your treatment, this specialist should be in close touch with your family doctor. It may be that while surgery takes place at a medical center, follow-up treatment, such as chemotherapy, can be administered in your family doctor's office under the medical oncologist's direction. More and more, physicians' offices and smaller hospitals can perform cancer follow-up care.

Finding Your Own Specialist

While you may trust your family doctor and his or her referral to various cancer specialists, it's important that the specialists and the places where they practice feel right to you.

In the event you don't feel well matched with the specialists you're referred to, or if your family doctor doesn't know who to refer you to, you may need to do some investigating on your own to find the best cancer specialists near you.

The best cancer specialists should be affiliated with

a national clinical research group. They should also be affiliated with one of the following:

1. A comprehensive cancer center. This is a designation given by the National Cancer Institute to facilities that receive grant support for, and systematically combine, laboratory research and clinical research.
2. A university.
3. A CCOP (Community Cooperative Outreach Program).
4. A CGOP (Cooperative Group Outreach Program).

These affiliations assure the patient that the specialist has access to the latest treatment information and has met rigid professional requirements for membership. They will also keep you away from frauds and charlatans.

If your doctor refers you to a specialist who does not belong to one of these, you should consider getting a second opinion before you agree to a treatment plan for your breast cancer.

Use the Library

The library can help you find the qualified surgeons and oncologists in your area. Most libraries carry two medical directories: *The Directory of Medical Specialists* and the *American Medical Association Directory*. You may also want to contact your local chapter of the American Cancer Society or the National Cancer Institute (see the Resources section at the end of the book) for other sources of names and information.

Is This the Right Specialist for You?

Once you have met with the specialist, consider whether the two of you are a good match. Doctors are people just like the rest of us. Some personalities mesh, and some clash. Like your family doctor, your medical oncologist and your surgeon(s) must be people you trust and can communicate with.

Some patients are conservative. So are some specialists. Other patients and specialists are more aggressive. Try to find specialists who are like you in this respect.

Also, if you feel excessively shy with a specialist or are intimidated by him or her, you're not going to be able to work as a team with that person in the crucially important journey you are embarking upon into the world of cancer treatment.

Try to Meet the Specialist First

If at all possible, arrange a consultation with the specialist before you decide on becoming his or her patient. Trust your instincts. Can you place your well-being in this person's hands? Here are some considerations:

- Does the specialist have a good reputation?
- When the specialist meets with you, does he or she show an interest in you and your feelings as well as in your disease?
- Does the specialist take time to explain things you don't understand well in language you can understand?

- Is the specialist direct with you, telling you exactly what will happen and what to expect?
- Does the specialist and his or her support staff treat you with courtesy and respect?

If you leave this first meeting feeling confident and positive, you've probably found a good match. If not, it will be worth the inconvenience and expense to talk to another specialist, in the event you have this option.

Sometimes there are no options. Depending on where you live, or on your financial circumstances, you may have no other choices. If this is the case, and if you trust this specialist, even though other factors such as communication may not be as satisfactory as you might like, you can work to strengthen the weak parts of your patient-doctor relationship and find it satisfactory.

How to Get the Best Treatment Possible

Finding the best medical personnel to help you in your recovery from cancer is an important step. Working effectively with them is another. It's not easy being a patient's ideal doctor. Nor is it easy being the ideal patient. Here are some tips:

When discussing your treatment with a specialist for the first time, ask to have time to get dressed after the exam before discussing treatment. That way you won't feel as vulnerable and you can feel more in charge of the situation. Most doctors are more comfortable with this as well.

Don't hesitate to bring a list of questions with you and to write down the doctor's answers. This shows that you're organized and thorough. To the doctor this says that you'll leave with the information you need and you won't forget it. Doctors appreciate working with patients who are informed and businesslike.

Don't, however, bring a tape recorder unless you've specifically requested this ahead of time and the doctor has assured you that it's fine. Most doctors find tape recorders very threatening, and the presence of one during your discussions will hamper open communication.

What Kind of Patient Gets the Best Care?

Physicians work best with:

Patients who stay calm. The doctors are on your side and want very much to help you. To do so, they need your full cooperation, and you can't give it to them if you are not in control of your emotions. Patients who are hostile or combative are very difficult to treat. Crying, however, is not only normal, but doctors expect it. They know how difficult this is for you.

If you are too upset to listen to what the doctor is telling you, say so. Usually you can take a break for a few minutes, or continue the consultation another day.

Patients who are organized. Doctors are busy people, and while they want to answer all your concerns and questions, it's important that you either have them written down or are prepared to ask them all at once in order to save time. Once your doctors know you won't waste their time, they'll more readily address all your concerns.

Patients who know their medical history. This may mean doing some checking before you come to the doctor's office. Medical personnel need an accurate history about you and your family. Your medical past can offer important clues about you.

It's very important that you never withhold information from your doctor. Sometimes patients are ashamed of something in their medical pasts and choose not to bring it up—when it could provide important clues for medical testing.

You need the results of your tests in hand. If you are going for a first-time consultation, carry your medical records and X rays with you or make sure ahead of time that they have arrived at the doctor's office.

Patients who are aware of their own bodies. Many women are sensitive enough to their own bodies that they know when something is working or when something isn't. They can often guide doctors by telling them of their suspicions or by reporting how they feel after a test. Doctors need this feedback. Sometimes patients act as though the doctor should know just how they feel. Doctors can only guess. If you hurt somewhere and don't say so, your doctor will not know and might overlook something important.

Patients who can communicate their needs. Again, doctors aren't mind readers. They appreciate patients who voice their concerns and who willingly respond to inquiries or directions from them. They need cooperation if they are to do their very best for you. There's no such thing as a "dumb" question. If it's something you want to know, then be sure to ask.

Even if you feel shy and tongue-tied, force yourself to talk to your doctor. It will get easier as time passes.

Remember that office nurses often know a great deal as well. You may be able to get many of your questions answered by the nurse, leaving you with fewer things to discuss with the doctor.

Patients who know what's going on. It's difficult for doctors to work with patients who never seem to understand what's happening. Often doctors will recommend books or articles to their patients to teach them about their illness. (Perhaps a doctor recommended this book to you.) And by paying close attention to what's happening to you, you can actually help your doctor, who may forget something about you or your treatment. Don't assume doctors remember everything. They don't—and they all appreciate being reminded.

One last thing. Ask your doctor if he or she has a time of day set aside for returning calls to patients. Many do. That way, you won't be trying to stay close to the phone all day, when the doctor may not plan to call you until late afternoon.

The Patient Advocate

One of the best things you can do for yourself is to bring someone with you to all your appointments with your doctor. This person will be your advocate and should be a trusted friend or relative.

Your advocate can take notes, give moral support during consultation and treatment, keep other people informed, help get you to appointments on time, and run interference with office and hospital personnel.

If you pick the right person, this can be a very successful arrangement for all concerned. Cancer treatment can be stressful, confusing, and sometimes, particularly when a new procedure is being started, downright scary. Your advocate can be a great help to you.

For an advocate to be a positive force rather than a detriment, this person must meet several requirements.

The advocate must feel comfortable with the medical profession. If you choose someone who is hostile, the physician will have to try to handle this, and in the process will take attention away from you.

Although it is extremely important for husbands or

lovers to be present when treatment options are discussed, they can be the worst advocates because they want medical professionals to do more for their loved ones than is often possible. If this person becomes a problem for medical personnel, it affects your care. Also, you may end up feeling guilty about this person's behavior.

The advocate must be someone you are comfortable with. Because you have cancer, you will have many areas of your body examined repeatedly. You don't want an advocate with you who is embarrassed by this or whose presence embarrasses you.

The advocate must have a flexible schedule. It can be tough enough for you to have to schedule appointments around job and family. If your advocate also has lots of responsibilities, he or she may not be able to be present when you need to have him or her with you.

The advocate must let you talk for yourself. The advocate situation doesn't work well when the advocate wants to talk for the patient. While this person is welcome to ask questions and encouraged to write down information for you, it's very important that you have direct contact with your medical team.

The Three of You

Ideally, medical personnel will talk to three people: you, your advocate, and your husband or lover. Your advocate is the least emotional of the three and the person charged with getting and understanding all information. Your loved one is there to give you moral and emotional support.

Except when there is a special circumstance, such as acute illness, request that family members or your advocate not call your doctors or attempt to make appointments with them to discuss your treatment plan or chances of cure without you present. Most doctors will consider this a breach of confidentiality. Even if the doctors know you or your family well, they will be reluctant to do this because it can be easily misconstrued as talking behind your back.

What If Your Doctor Won't Listen to You?

Challenging a physician is almost always difficult for a patient. After all, this is the expert, the person who went to medical school, right? But it's your body, and you may have a better grasp of what's happening to it than the doctor has. Patients often sense that something is wrong with them long before a doctor can find the problem.

The difficulty of challenging an expert is the possibility of straining your relationship and making both of you uncomfortable. But there are ways to do it that can keep your relationship strong.

Say, for example, that you have a lump in your breast that the doctor thinks is a benign cyst. You would feel better having a biopsy done in order to know for sure what it is. You could confront the doctor by saying, "I don't think you're right. Biopsy this lump."

But a more diplomatic, and thus a better way would be to say, "I know you're probably right, but I'm feeling really nervous about this. Please do a biopsy so I can have peace of mind."

Let Your Needs Be Known

What you must do is let the doctor and the office staff know what you need, what kind of person you are, and your individual preferences. Speak up.

If you want a private instead of a semiprivate hospital room, let the staff know *before* the arrangements are made.

Perhaps watching blood withdrawn makes you anxious or even light-headed. Ask if you could lie down, turning your head away so you don't have to see the procedure.

If you would prefer one nurse over another when you're receiving treatment, let someone know. You should find the office staff accommodating of your requests, as long as they are reasonable.

The Hurried Doctor

The doctor who's always in a hurry is also troublesome to patients. You have so much you need to ask, and such great need for comforting, but you feel guilty taking the doctor's time. How do you slow down a person like this?

First, remind yourself that you have a right to a reasonable amount of the doctor's time. However, if a doctor must spend an extended amount of time answering your questions to your satisfaction, you may be billed for it. To prevent this, don't ask the same questions over and over. Some patients do this, hoping to get a different answer—one they would prefer. Medicine doesn't work this way.

Some insurance plans will only reimburse the doctor for a certain amount regardless of the amount of time spent with a patient. If your doctors must constantly spend much more time with you in order to answer the same questions over and over, they naturally won't be happy about this.

If you know that you have a lot of questions you need to have answered, mention this when you are making your appointment so the staff will know to allot extra time for you. You may even need to make an extra appointment just to ask questions.

Remember, too, that the office nurse or a nurse clinician can often answer your questions. Take advantage of this.

The Ideal Patient-Doctor Relationship

Some patients want to take a more active role in their treatment than others. A few patients want virtually no role at all. They want the doctor to make all decisions for them. At the other extreme are those few who want to make all the decisions, yet they still hold the physician accountable for their well-being, even if something negative happens because of their decision.

In the best relationship, the doctor presents alternatives to the patient, and together they decide on the best course of treatment. Patients who are actively involved in this decision-making process tend to do the best.

Everyone's heard the stories about the patient who was told she had six months to live. Since the doctor told her this, she believed it. She set her affairs in order and in six months she was dead. Then there's the patient told she has six months to live who says, "No. I refuse to die." And years later she's alive and well.

It's not that living or dying is a choice. But your attitude about your illness and what *you* intend to do about it—in conjunction with your medical treatment team—can be a key factor in your treatment tolerance and recovery.

Questions to Ask Your Doctor

When you first find out you have breast cancer, you're probably too much in shock to ask many questions. In fact, it may not be until you've already been referred to a cancer specialist that you have an opportunity to ask what's on your mind.

Here are some things you will want to know about the general course of your disease and treatment:

- What can you tell at this point about my breast cancer?
- Are additional tests needed before an optimal treatment plan can be recommended?
- If not, what kind of treatment do you recommend?
- Does it have immediate side effects?
- What are the long-term risks of this treatment?
- Will I be able to continue working during treatment?
- Where will I go for treatment?
- How long does it take?
- How much does it cost?
- What are reasonable alternative treatments, if any?
- If you are performing surgery, what will I look like afterward?

When selecting a cancer specialist to direct your treatment, consider the following questions:

- Is he/she highly qualified and/or recommended? Does he or she have a university, comprehensive cancer center, CCOP, or CGOP affiliation?
- Is the office staff courteous and friendly?
- Am I comfortable with the doctor?
- Does he or she take time to answer my questions and discuss my options?

Finally, here are the two most important questions:

- Does the doctor seem to care about me as a person?
- Do I feel confident entrusting my health care to this doctor?

3 How Your Cancer Was Discovered and Diagnosed

At the time your breast cancer was discovered and diagnosed, you may have been in such emotional turmoil that you were unsure what doctors were telling you.

When we are under stress—and this is certainly one of the most stressful of situations—our minds tend to freeze up, allowing us to absorb only as much information as we need moment to moment to get along. It's a protective device, and a good one, but it means that later, when we're trying to remember what we've been told about something, we can't recall everything that was said to us.

A review of what's been going on may be helpful.

*   *   *

Discovering Your Cancer

Women discover 90 percent of the lumps in their breasts through self-examination. While a lump or thickening in the breast or under the arm is the most common symptom of breast cancer, maybe you became concerned about nipple discharge, or a change in the size or shape of one of your breasts, or you noticed a change in the color or texture of your breast skin or nipple.

It's also possible that your family doctor found a suspicious lump or thickening during your annual exam. Or perhaps something suspicious was noted when you had a mammogram.

Your initial reaction might have been that nothing could be wrong with you because the lump or thickness was not painful. Cysts, which are harmless, often hurt because they are influenced by hormonal cycles in your body. But as you now know, cancerous lumps are usually painless. Cancers have a gritty, hard feel and a rough texture. Cysts are often smooth and firm.

Mammography

At the time you report a suspicious lump or thickening to your doctor, you may be asked to get a mammogram before your appointment—even if you've recently had one.

A mammogram produces a detailed image that can reveal abnormalities in the breasts. The resulting picture is read by a *radiologist*—a physician with special training in X-ray diagnostics. (See Illustration #3.)

Some women worry about X-ray exposure during

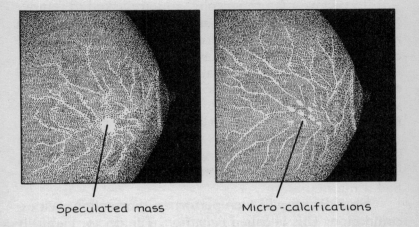

Speculated mass   Micro-calcifications

illustration 3: A mammogram can reveal many problems before they can be felt. The radiologist who reads a mammogram looks for three signs of cancer: (1) an irregular crablike mass, as in the left illustration; (2) microcalcifications, as in the right illustration; or (3) a thickening in the skin.

mammography. But new techniques involve such minute amounts of radiation that the benefits vastly outweigh any risks.

To receive mammography, you are asked to remove your clothing to the waist and put on a cotton drape. A female technologist positions one breast at a time against the X-ray machine and takes the X rays.

The entire procedure takes only a few minutes and most women think it is painless. A few complain about discomfort while the breast is being compressed against the machine in order to get a clear reading.

Palpation and Aspiration

Your doctor will then perform a thorough breast examination. This is called *palpation*. The doctor carefully feels the breast, trying to determine the lump or thickening's size, texture, and whether or not it is movable.

To determine if a lump is cancerous, the next step is usually *aspiration*. This procedure sounds more scary than it actually is. You either sit up or lie down, depending on which position offers the doctor best access to the lump. The doctor injects some local anesthetic into the area and, when it is numb, inserts a long, fine needle with a syringe on the end into the lump or mass. (See Illustration #4.)

When a suspicious area is a cyst, the fluid that is extracted may vary in color from clear to green, red, or blue. The color has no significance. The area painlessly disappears as the fluid is withdrawn. If it does not, then it's a solid mass—a tumor—which may or may not be cancerous. Eighty percent are not cancerous.

When a mass is not palpable but is visible on mammography, then needle aspiration or a needle or wire-

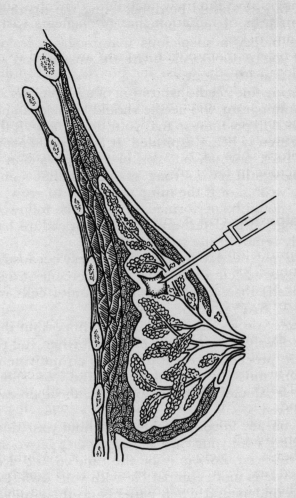

illustration 4: During needle aspiration, a fine needle is inserted into the breast mass to draw out cells and/or fluid to be examined microscopically.

guided biopsy should be done, using the mammogram to position the needle or wire. If your doctor doesn't plan to biopsy a suspicious mammogram lesion, ask why. If you're not satisfied with the answer you receive, request that it be done.

During fine needle aspiration of a suspicious area on the mammogram, the needle should be placed and photographed in position so that your doctor *knows* that the correct area is being aspirated. If this needle aspiration comes back normal, but you or your physician or the radiologist still have strong suspicions that something may be wrong, or if the lump continues to grow, then a biopsy should be performed. It should be followed by a mammogram to determine that the procedure has successfully removed the suspicious area.

You may need to insist on the biopsy because needle aspirates are accurate only 85 to 90 percent of the time. This means that, using aspiration, tumor cells may be missed 10 to 15 percent of the time.

While you should insist, it's also important that you not needlessly alienate your physician when you request a certain procedure. Each patient is an individual, and treatment must be individualized. But you should be given a satisfactory explanation if the above precautions aren't taken.

If you are uncomfortable with how your doctor is proceeding with your care, and you can't get your questions answered, now may be the time to find a doctor whose style is more compatible with your own. Doctors truly do understand when patients do this—and would advise you to do it if you or your family members are uncomfortable.

Other Diagnostic Procedures

In the event that your breasts are especially fibrous and it's difficult to get a clear picture of them using mammography, your doctor may recommend one of the following procedures:

Ultrasound, where high-frequency sound waves are used to map the internal structures of the breast to help determine whether a lump is a cyst or solid mass. This test is generally used *along with* mammography.

Thermography, a rarely used test that measures minute heat patterns in the breasts to detect abnormalities.

CAT scan, a procedure sometimes used with women for whom mammography is not helpful because of the presence of severe fibrocystic disease.

Make Sure You're Convinced

No matter what the result of these testing procedures, if you're not convinced that the results are accurate, *trust your instincts* and request that more or different testing be done.

All of these tests are fallible. As we've stressed before, you know your body best, you have the most at stake here, and you need to have as much diagnosis as it takes to convince you and your doctors that results are accurate.

The Diagnostic Biopsy

A diagnostic biopsy is the removal of tissue cells from the breast mass to determine if it's cancerous. Some doctors perform the biopsy in their offices using local anesthetic, and some want patients to check into the hospital and to be asleep with general anesthetic.

Typically, small tumors can be removed in a doctor's office or the outpatient department of a hospital using local anesthesia. During this procedure, the area is numbed. You are awake, but feel no pain.

If your tumor is very large or located quite deep in the breast—or if those factors are not known—a doctor is more likely to want to remove it in the hospital with you asleep.

When a doctor performs an *incisional biopsy,* only part of the suspicious mass is removed for analysis. When the entire mass is removed, it's called an *excisional biopsy.*

You'll want to have an excisional rather than an incisional biopsy if possible so there is little risk of cancerous cells from the remaining mass being knocked loose and finding their way into the bloodstream. Once again, if your doctor or surgeon doesn't plan to do this, *find out why.*

The Key Words Are "Flash-Frozen"

The most important factor in determining where the biopsy takes place—a hospital or a doctor's office—is that cancerous biopsied material *must be* immediately flash-frozen in liquid nitrogen so that all information needed can eventually be obtained from it. This is the only chance there will be to get this information, so this is very important. Use of frozen tissue is currently the most accurate way of testing for hormone receptors and the rate of tumor growth.

By viewing the *frozen section,* the pathologist can usually tell very quickly if cancer is present. More thorough testing requires more time, so part of the tissue removed is subjected to a *permanent section.* As part of this procedure, tissue is "fixed" by a special procedure so it won't decompose, embedded in a waxy substance, and then cut into sections, stained, and placed on slides so the pathologist and your doctor can look at it under a microscope. Cellular detail is better on permanent section than frozen section. It is always possible that the diagnosis can change after permanent section.

The Two-Step Biopsy

As a rule, doctors today perform a biopsy, and if cancer is found and surgery recommended, they may wait as long as two weeks to do it. (Studies show that this wait has no negative impact on the outcome of your surgery.)

Many things happen during that time. You must decide on the right course of treatment for you. You may want to visit with one or more radiation oncologists and breast cancer surgeons to talk about breast sparing procedures. Perhaps you'll want to talk to a plastic surgeon about breast reconstruction. If your tumor is large or has other negative features and the surgeon suspects you will need follow-up chemotherapy and/or hormone therapy, you may also want to consult a medical oncologist.

Also, as we've mentioned, it takes one to two weeks

for the more complicated tests to be completed on the cancerous tissue. These tests tell doctors how fast the cancer is growing and whether it might respond best to hormone therapy or chemotherapy.

You will want to meet with your physician and/or oncologist to discuss lumpectomy and the various types of mastectomies in order to determine the best procedure for you.

You also need time to make preparations at home and/or work in order to be out of commission for a while during the initial stages of recovery from surgery and follow-up treatment.

Finally, you need time to adjust to the shock of finding out you have cancer before you can begin your recovery.

The One-Step Biopsy and Mastectomy

Occasionally doctors still recommend that patients have a combination of a biopsy and a mastectomy all at one time. There are some good reasons for this.

For some women, because of poor health or because general anesthesia poses a particular risk to them, the one-step method is safer.

These women will want to discuss all options with their surgeons before the biopsy, and then consent to having an immediate mastectomy, all in one operation, in the event cancer is found.

A patient may already know she has cancer because of a prior aspirate, and she wants everything taken care of immediately.

It Must Be Your Decision

Unless there are health problems involved, whether to have the one-step or two-step procedure should be your decision. But so many important things happen in that time period between the biopsy and the surgery that, whenever possible, we recommend the two-step biopsy.

What the Biopsy Reveals About Your Cancer

The biopsy will enable the pathologist to tell whether or not the lump in your breast is malignant. Twenty percent of biopsied lumps are. The biopsy also allows other information to be obtained that will guide your medical team in putting together the best treatment plan for you.

Odd as it may sound, some tumors are more malignant than others. (The word "malignant" comes from "malign," which literally means "evil.") Viewing the biopsy specimen will help determine how aggressive the tumor is, if it has invaded outside the duct or lobule from which it arose, and if it has invaded the breast lymphatic vessels and/or the blood vessels.

The three most important things to know in order to predict whether your tumor might recur is (1) how many lymph nodes have been invaded by the cancer, (2) the size of the tumor, and (3) how fast the tumor is growing. Finding out if your tumor reacts to hormones also helps determine the correct treatment for you.

The biopsy does not reveal whether your lymph

49

nodes are involved. This information is obtained from the axillary dissection and is explained in Chapter Four.

Some of the Terms You Will Be Hearing

You may become frustrated by all the medical terminology you will hear at the time your cancer is being discovered and diagnosed, but your understanding of the following five terms is important. They refer to tests that will assist your doctors in determining what kind of surgery and treatment you will need. Here are very basic explanations:

Ploidy is a measurement of the amount of genetic material that helps predict how the tumor will behave.

S-phase refers to a measurement of how fast the tumor is growing.

Epidermal growth factor receptors indirectly measure how fast the tumor is growing. They can help predict how you might respond to hormone therapy, along with the hormone receptor tests.

Her-II-neu is the name of an oncogene that is often associated with a poor prognosis. An *oncogene* is a gene in a cell that probably helps regulate cell growth and division. When it is uncontrolled, it may help turn a normal cell into a cancerous one. If tests reveal a high number of oncogene-directed proteins in the cancer cells, this may be an indicator that the cancer is more likely to recur and should be treated aggressively.

Cathepsin D is an enzyme present in breast tissue and in other cells that helps break down tissue. Large amounts of this enzyme in breast tissue may indicate a high degree of invasion into surrounding healthy tissue.

Estrogen Receptor Tests

One of the most important tests you will hear about is the estrogen receptor test. To understand the importance of this test, think of the cellular hormone receptors and the hormones in your breasts as locks and keys.

The hormone receptor is a lock, and the hormone is a key. When they come together, the hormone key can turn the hormone receptor lock. When the lock is turned, genetic material (DNA) is activated. This activated DNA then signals the cell to initiate an appropriate function, such as to start growing, or to make milk.

In a normal breast, the combining of cell receptors and hormones happens at a natural, cyclical pace. At certain times of life—for example, during pregnancy and lactation—there is an increase in the pace at which cell receptors and hormones combine, and the subsequent cell growth speeds up. But then, following pregnancy and lactation, when it's time for the pace to slow, it does.

In a cancerous breast, however, the mechanism for speeding up and slowing the pace of cell function and division may get messed up. Balance is often lost. The receptors or "locks" for hormones may be overproduced by the cancer cell, allowing cancer growth to be stimulated by the estrogen (female hormone) normally in your body.

If the tumor produces too much hormone receptor, your tumor is said to be *estrogen receptor positive*. In this case, part of your treatment may involve removing estrogen from your body. This can be done through pills, injections, or by removing your ovaries.

So hormone receptor tests help your doctors determine whether cancer cells might be destroyed or slowed by administering anti-estrogens or other antihormones, or if administering chemotherapy will be more effective.

Treatment of Tumors

Fast-growing tumors are usually ER (estrogen receptor) negative, and surgery is followed by chemotherapy.

Slow-growing tumors are often ER positive and may be best treated with hormonal intervention. This may be with an anti-estrogen pill called tamoxifen. In premenopausal women, this may also include removal of the ovaries in order to stop production of estrogen, or use of an injection called Zoladex, which suppresses pituitary stimulation of estrogen release by the ovaries. ER positive patients shouldn't be given long-term estrogen supplements in any form.

If a premenopausal ER positive patient receives chemotherapy as part of her treatment, and if she's still menstruating at the end of her chemotherapy treatment (chemotherapy often causes ovarian damage and a drop in the body's estrogen), she may also need antihormonal treatment to further suppress any remaining cancer cells.

Even if an ER positive patient has already gone through menopause, she may still have estrogen in her body because the liver, fat cells, and breast tissue can also produce estrogen. She will also need antihormone treatment. In this instance, treatment will probably include taking an anti-estrogen drug, such as tamoxifen.

*   *   *

Predicting Recurrence

Yet another reason why the hormone receptor test is important is that it is one of the many prognostic factors that help determine if a patient is at risk for recurrence of cancer. We now know that women whose cells are estrogen receptor *negative* are at a higher risk of early recurrence of cancer than are women who are estrogen receptor *positive.*

Why is this so? Probably because negative receptor tumors often grow faster than positive receptor tumors.

The Stages of Cancer

The earliest stage of breast cancer is called *carcinoma in situ.* In this stage, the cancer is totally within the duct and has not spread into surrounding breast tissue.

In *Stage I* breast cancer, the tumor is very small (usually less than an inch in length). It has invaded breast tissue outside the ducts but has not spread outside the breast and does not involve the lymph glands under the arm. When the lymph glands are not involved, the tumor is referred to as *node negative.*

In *Stage II,* the tumor may be up to two inches in length. The lymph glands may or may not be involved, but there's no evidence that the cancer has spread elsewhere in the body.

Early Stage Is Highly Curable

These early stages of breast cancer are considered the most curable because the cancer is located only in the breast and possibly the nodes, but has not spread to other parts of the body.

Usually patients with early-stage breast cancer undergo surgery and sometimes radiation therapy. Chemotherapy and/or hormone therapy may be given if doctors suspect there's at least a 30 percent chance that the tumor may eventually show up somewhere else in the body.

In *Stage III* breast cancer, the tumor may be quite large—more than two inches in length—the lymph nodes are usually involved, and the cancer may invade the skin or muscles of the chest wall. In Stage III, there is no evidence that cancer has spread to distant organs.

Treatment for Stage III patients may begin with chemotherapy to shrink the mass, followed by mastectomy or lumpectomy, and then more chemotherapy and often radiation as well. Today, Stage III breast cancer is being treated more aggressively than it has been in the past, and the outlook for cure is improving.

Stage IV patients are those whose breast cancer has spread to at least one organ of the body. Usually it is the brain, liver, bones, or lungs. Treatment usually consists of trying to shrink the tumor with hormone therapy, chemotherapy, and radiation. Such treatment is successful in inducing remission in 50 to 80 percent of all cases. Many factors, including a woman's general health, influence the final outcome of treatment. Complete cure is rare in Stage IV disease, but some women live for ten to twenty years with it and enjoy relatively normal lives.

The Spread of Breast Cancer

The growth of breast cancer can differ dramatically from person to person and may also change as the tumor evolves. Anywhere from 1 percent to 60 percent of the cancer cells can be growing at any given time. If the cells are growing very fast, they may spread to other organs of the body through the bloodstream or via the lymph nodes before a lump or mass is detected in the breast. Sometimes, because the cancer has spread to the bone early in the course of the disease, back pain is the first sign that anything is wrong.

Once the underarm lymph nodes are involved, chances increase dramatically that the cancer cells have found their way into the bloodstream and have seeded other organs.

Lymph Node Involvement

The pathologist can determine how many lymph nodes are involved from an axillary (underarm) lymph node dissection procedure. This may be done on its own or as part of a mastectomy.

If four or more nodes are positive for cancer, then chances are 50 to 75 percent that the cancer cells have escaped to the rest of the body.

The rule of thumb is that the fewer the number of nodes involved, the better the outlook and the shorter the duration of treatment. The type and aggressiveness of the treatment is determined by the rapidity of growth, as well as by other factors, including how abnormal the cancer cells appear and the results of the hormone receptor tests.

What Comes Next

Once cancer is diagnosed, your doctor will probably order a series of tests, all of which will help determine your general health and any possibility of the spread of cancer in your system. These tests may include:

- Urinalysis.
- Blood tests to measure liver and bone function.
- Liver scan.
- Bone scan.
- Chest X ray.
- Gynecological exam to rule out spread of cancer to the ovaries.

Questions to Ask Your Doctor

Before and after your biopsy you will have many questions for your doctor. Remember that your advocate can help you record the answers to the questions you ask so you can remember what your doctors tell you. Keep careful notes, for you are likely to refer back to them many times. Here are some of the things you may want to ask:

- Can I have a "biopsy only" at this time?
- What kind of biopsy—incisional or excisional—are you going to perform and why?
- What kinds of tests will be performed on the bi-

opsy, other than looking in the microscope to see if I have cancer?

- Are you going to freeze a portion of the tumor? If not, why not?
- How soon will you have the results and when will I get them?
- How and where will you perform the biopsy?
- What type of anesthesia (local or general) will you use, and why?

4 Treatment Options

Usually, the diagnosis of breast cancer means surgery. Trying to understand surgical options and selecting the right one for you is no easy matter when you must also cope with the shock of learning you have cancer and now face an operation.

But it's important that you understand each of the surgical options and some of the factors that bear on selecting one over another. Because it's only possible here to discuss them in general terms, you'll want to question your doctor carefully about the right surgery for you.

Such factors as your overall health, age, health history, cell type, the size of tumor involved, what stage your cancer is in, and what, if any, additional treatment you will need after surgery will influence this decision. Be sure to be open-minded and to listen carefully to your doctor's advice. What worked for a neighbor, relative, or the friend of a friend will not necessarily be the best approach for you.

Types of Surgery

For almost a century, prevailing medical thinking was that the more extensive the surgery for breast cancer, the greater were the chances for recovery.

Radical Mastectomy

Even into the 1970s, most doctors felt the radical mastectomy, also called the Halsted radical in honor of the doctor who developed it, was the only advisable procedure when breast cancer was found.

William Halsted was an American surgeon affiliated with Johns Hopkins medical school and hospital in the late 1800s. It was Halsted's belief that breast cancer started at a central point in the breast and gradually spread outward in a systematic fashion into surrounding tissue and lymph nodes and then into the rest of the body.

Because he didn't place as much emphasis on the role of the blood supply in carrying cancer cells to the rest of the body, he felt that the greatest chance for recovery lay in removing the entire breast, the underlying chest muscles, and the underarm lymph nodes.

In Halsted's day, surgery was the only type of treatment available for breast cancer. Hospitals were dreaded places where people often died. Anesthetic techniques were poor. Consequently, by the time a physician resorted to surgery to try to save a patient, tumors were usually quite large. Halsted's technique gave patients the greatest chance of survival.

Treatment Has Changed

Today we know that breast cancer often spreads in its earliest stages—usually through the blood vessels—to other organs. The lymph nodes and surrounding breast tissue do not need to be involved for this to occur. Radical surgery, which removes surrounding breast tissue, chest muscles, and lymph nodes, will not increase the cure rate if tumor cells have already spread to other organs via the blood vessels before surgery takes place.

The only time a radical mastectomy is recommended today is in the case of very large tumors to improve local control. Fortunately, this is a rare occurrence. Removing a large amount of normal tissue around the breast will not improve the cure rate if the chances are high that the tumor has already spread through the bloodstream. But in instances where there is little concern that the tumor has spread throughout the body, the cure rate is much more closely connected with adequate removal of the tumor—and more radical surgery has the best chance of doing that.

Fortunately, in the case of small tumors, less radical surgery is required for local control. (See Illustration #5.)

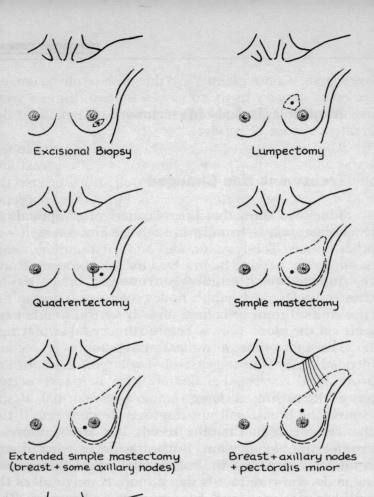

Excisional Biopsy

Lumpectomy

Quadrentectomy

Simple mastectomy

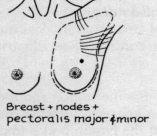

Extended simple mastectomy
(breast + some axillary nodes)

Breast + axillary nodes
+ pectoralis minor

Breast + nodes +
pectoralis major & minor

illustration 5: Breast cancer surgery offers a variety of options
today that weren't available in the past. The outlined areas
show the section of breast removed in each type of surgery.

Modified Radical Mastectomy

This is the most common surgical procedure in use today. As with the Halsted mastectomy, the breast and underarm lymph nodes are removed. But because the major chest wall muscles are left intact, breast reconstruction is facilitated, and, with physical rehabilitation, the patient will regain full use of her arm(s).

Simple or Total Mastectomy

While the entire breast is removed in a simple mastectomy, none or only a few of the underarm lymph nodes are taken for examination.

Partial Mastectomy

This procedure is also called a quadrantectomy. It removes the tumor along with a large amount of surrounding healthy tissue, some of the muscle lining, and some overlying skin. As a precaution, some or all of the lymph nodes are often removed at the same time. This latter procedure is call an *axillary dissection*.

Lumpectomy

This procedure removes just the tumor and a minimum of surrounding tissue. A separate incision may be used to remove some or all of the lymph nodes (axillary dissection). Radiation treatment follow-up is a necessity when lumpectomy is used—a consideration in deciding if lumpectomy is a good choice for a woman.

Deciding on the Best Surgery for You

With so many options, deciding on which type of surgery is best for you can be complicated. Trust your doctor's guidance. Remember, your medical history, age, the size of your breast, the stage of your cancer, the size of the tumor, your distance from a good radiation facility, the type of postoperative chemo or hormone therapy you might need, *and your preferences* are all important considerations.

You need to feel that the surgery you choose is right for you.

Sometimes doctors offer no options, determining that a certain type of surgery is, under the circumstances, the best choice. Again, trust your doctor, but ask *why* this choice is best. Before you agree to it, make sure you're clear on what is going to be done and why.

If you don't feel comfortable with what you're being told, you'll be happier in the long run if you seek out a second opinion.

Surgery Advantages and Disadvantages

Each type of surgery has its advantages and disadvantages. Here are some general guidelines. (See Illustration #6.)

Radical mastectomy: With newer methods of surgery, radiation, and chemotherapy, the Halsted radical mastectomy is useful today only if the breast cancer has invaded the underlying chest muscles. This may have

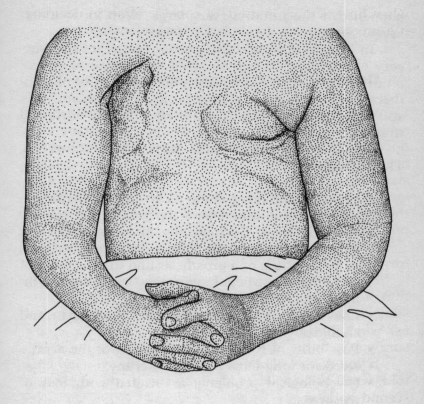

illustration 6: Reconstruction can be difficult after a radical mastectomy because so much underlying muscle and tissue has been removed (area on left side of the illustration). With a modified radical or extended simple mastectomy (area on right side of illustration), results are much better. There is less chance of arm swelling and more tissue remains on the chest wall, allowing a normal upper chest contour.

happened if the tumor is very large, deep, or is ulcerating.

In historical perspective, during the years this surgery was popular, it helped avoid recurrence of cancer on the chest wall at a time when no radiation or chemotherapy was available to help avoid that problem. It is still useful today in treatment of large locally advanced tumors.

The disadvantages of this surgery are numerous. They include:

- Leaving behind a long scar and a flattened, sunken chest wall where the breast and muscle formerly were. Cosmetically, this means a poor appearance, with little chance for reconstruction.
- Difficult fitting of a prosthesis and the necessity of specially constructed swimsuits and other clothing items.
- Loss of strength and some use of the arm and shoulder.
- Possibility of *lymphedema* (swelling of the arm).
- Need for long-term physical therapy.
- Psychological problems associated with loss of the breast.

Modified radical or simple mastectomies: The modified radical and the simple mastectomy with axillary dissection have several advantages. These include:

- Ability to have the surgery performed in almost any hospital, thus allowing for treatment near home.
- Option of having reconstructive surgery.
- Ease of fitting a prosthesis.
- Little or no loss of arm strength.

- Fairly normal upper chest contour.
- Little or no arm swelling.

Note: If your doctor recommends having one of these types of mastectomies, discuss the option of breast reconstruction before the surgery. It may affect the kind of incision used by the surgeon. Reconstruction is easier if the incision is horizontal.

In some instances, reconstruction can even be performed at the time of the mastectomy. In most instances, it will be performed after all treatment is completed.

Disadvantages of the modified radical or simple mastectomies include:

- Possible swelling, long- or short-term, under the arm.
- Possible need for physical therapy.
- Psychological problems with the loss of the breast.

Partial mastectomy or lumpectomy: When the breast is kept intact, the major disadvantage is:

- Radiation treatments must be given daily for five to six weeks. Radiation can cause damage to the skin, esophagus (swallowing tube), heart, and lungs. In many radiation treatment facilities, however, sophisticated computerized treatment planning and the use of several different types of radiation minimize normal tissue damage.
- With lumpectomy there is a higher chance of recurrence of breast cancer in the breast or chest wall area than with mastectomy.

However, the advantages of this type of surgery are important:

- The breast and nipple are basically unchanged, usually giving the best overall cosmetic appearance.
- Muscle loss and follow-up problems with the arm or shoulder are minimal.
- Because the breast is intact (although usually not completely normal) there are fewer postsurgical psychological problems than with mastectomies. Most women who undergo this type of treatment report good to excellent cosmetic results, and the appearance of the breast can have significant impact on how a woman feels about herself.

Mastectomies versus Lumpectomies

Women's magazines have run numerous articles lately relating stories that go something like this: A woman finds out she has breast cancer and her doctor recommends a mastectomy. She protests, insisting she won't allow her breast to be removed. She finds a doctor who agrees to do a lumpectomy. She bitterly tells her story, accusing the medical community of advising unnecessary mutilation of women.

When such stories appear in the popular press, doctors are inundated with calls from patients, their friends, and family members questioning the value of an impending or previously performed mastectomy. Doctors must then try to explain what the articles didn't—that lumpectomies are appropriate only when certain criteria are met.

Studies indicate that long-term survival rates for patients receiving lumpectomies-plus-radiation are equal to those for patients receiving mastectomies in early-stage cancer. Note the words "early stage." In more advanced cancer (Stage III or IV) mastectomy is still the most appropriate treatment because usually it is the only way to adequately remove the tumor from the chest wall.

In early-stage cancer, a variety of factors help determine the best treatment option.

Medical Considerations

Lumpectomy for invasive breast cancer always requires radiation to help kill undetected cancer cells that may still be present in the breast. In a woman with poor heart or lung function, radiation of the chest might cause serious problems since some radiation usually penetrates to these organs. Potential heart damage is a particular concern when the left breast is involved because the heart is on the left.

Patients with multifocal breast cancer have several distinct areas where the cancer has started. They do better with mastectomies than lumpectomies.

Mastectomy may also be better than lumpectomy and radiation in a patient with a 20 percent or greater risk of developing cancer in the other breast. These patients have either a strong family history of breast cancer, multifocal cancer, or lobular carcinoma in situ in the affected breast. They might want to consider mastectomy with later removal of the tissue from the remaining breast, along with bilateral reconstruction.

Finally, it's important that the patient be close to a treatment facility with a radiation oncologist and support personnel skilled in postlumpectomy treatment planning and administration. The treatment program must be administered daily for five to six weeks. If radiotherapists experienced in this procedure are not available in your area, mastectomy with immediate or delayed reconstruction may be the better choice for you.

Even if you have access to outstanding care, the cost and inconvenience of such extensive treatment can be a factor in deciding whether to have a lumpectomy.

Cosmetic Considerations

Lumpectomies for tumors over two inches in size often do not give satisfactory cosmetic results. The loss of breast volume and the follow-up radiation can cause scarring and retraction of the skin. There are programs in which chemotherapy is administered first in order to make lumpectomy possible. These are still considered experimental.

Large-breasted women face an additional risk: They may end up with breasts noticeably different in size.

Skin elasticity is also an important consideration. Elderly women with poor skin elasticity may find they have asymmetrical breasts after treatment. Sometimes younger women don't have good skin elasticity, either, and this is an important factor in determining whether the cosmetic results of lumpectomy will be satisfactory.

The Ideal Candidate

In general, the ideal candidate for lumpectomy with radiation is a small-breasted woman with good skin elasticity and a primary tumor two inches or less in diameter. If you are not this ideal candidate, this is probably not the right surgical option for you.

Psychological Considerations

We'll talk at length in later chapters about the psychological repercussions of breast cancer. For now, try to think carefully about how you will feel about each of these types of surgery. Sometimes women suffer from severe depression after they undergo a modified radical mastectomy. Some feel they are no longer complete women because their femininity was closely tied to their breasts.

If you feel this way, try to discuss your concerns with your doctor, the nursing staff, a trusted friend or loved one, or another woman who has had a mastectomy before you undergo your surgery. Starting to work through your fears and concerns *before* you lose a breast will help your emotional recovery after the fact.

How you feel will also have a strong bearing on whether you opt for reconstructive surgery. And this issue, too, should be thoroughly discussed before your surgery if you're going to have a mastectomy.

Questions to Ask Your Doctor

- Which surgical options are appropriate for me?
- Which one do you recommend and why?
- What are the potential risks and benefits of this option?
- Am I a candidate for any other procedure?

- If so, what are the risks and benefits of this alternative?

Once you've selected a type of surgery, ask:

- How is this surgery performed?
- How much time will I spend in the hospital?

5 What Happens When You Go to the Hospital for Surgery

The prospect of major surgery frightens most people. Worry and fear of the unknown can be worse than the actual experience.

While each hospital has its own policies and procedures, many things will be similar. What follows is a description, in general terms, of what you can expect.

What Happens Prior to Surgery

In the past, patients always checked into the hospital the day before their surgery. Now this rule varies, depending on your health, your insurance, and the hospital. You may be asked to check into the hospital the afternoon before, the evening before, or you may come to the hospital the morning of your surgery.

No matter when you check in, for security reasons, don't bring jewelry or valuables with you to the hospital. Also, don't wear any fingernail polish. The medical staff will be checking your fingertips to assist in monitoring your vital signs during surgery, and polish gets in the way.

If you do not stay in the hospital the night before your surgery, you will be instructed not to eat anything after midnight. If you know that sleeping that night will be difficult for you, consider asking your doctor for a sleeping pill or relaxant to help you. It's possible that you will be instructed to shower with an antibacterial soap and shave your underarms before you come to the hospital.

If you check in the morning of your surgery, you will probably visit the hospital several days ahead of time for blood and urine tests and a chest X ray. Then again, some hospitals do these just before surgery.

Meeting the Anesthesiologist

At some point before your surgery, whether it's several days ahead when you come for tests, the night before, or the morning of surgery, your anesthesiologist will meet with you. This is the doctor who administers the medication (anesthesia) that puts you to sleep during your operation. He or she needs to know certain things about you and will ask you a series of questions. These will relate to your medical history, past experience with anesthesia, and allergies. You'll also be asked if you are taking any medications and if you have experienced any heart, lung, or kidney problems. You'll also be asked if you have had any difficulty with anesthesia during any previous surgery.

Whether or not you smoke is also important to the anesthesiologist. Smoking irritates the airways and may cause heart and lung damage. Also, smokers have higher carbon monoxide levels in their blood. Prior knowledge of these factors is important in order to administer anesthesia safely.

You've probably answered all these questions before for other medical personnel, but the anesthesiologist needs this information for different reasons. In order for you to receive the best care possible, your thoroughness, patience, and understanding in answering all inquiries is important.

Surgical Preparation

If you check in the morning of your surgery, you will go to the surgery admitting area. You will be asked to sign consent forms stating that you understand the surgery you are going to have as well as the risks involved with it.

If your husband, lover, or a friend is with you, they can usually stay while you sign forms or meet with the anesthesiologist, but then you will have to say good-bye to them and a nurse will take you to a changing area where you will put on a hospital gown.

Many hospitals have a policy of assigning one nurse to one or two patients at a time, and this person stays with you or checks in frequently with you during this preliminary period before surgery begins. Whether there is one nurse or several, there will be someone who takes a special interest in you and will look after your needs.

75

Let Your Needs Be Known

Whether you are working with one staff nurse or several during this initial period, be sure to make your needs known and to ask whatever questions you have. In addition to their knowledge, these nurses understand that you may have many questions or concerns because they have worked with many patients about to go into surgery. They can be very helpful to you if you will let them.

Once you have changed into a hospital gown, you will be asked to lie down on a hospital gurney, which looks sort of like a cot on wheels.

The Holding Area

The holding area will probably be a big room with curtained-off sections. You will wait in one of these until you go to surgery. While you are in the holding area, an IV will be started. An IV is a solution of sugar and mineral water that drips into a vein in your hand or arm to keep you from becoming dehydrated or developing low blood sugar during surgery. The anesthesia or any other medication will be administered through this solution.

The Surgical Suite

When you are being wheeled into the surgery suite, you may be surprised by how cool the temperature feels. The cool temperature aids in infection control. In addition to the coolness, the room will be bright and very clean. All of the medical personnel will wear sterile masks, hats, gloves, and loose-fitting pants and tops called "scrubs." Because of all this clothing, you may not recognize your surgeon or anesthesiologist.

There may or may not be piped-in music. Some surgeons want it and some don't. Of those who do, many select their own music. Usually it's something light and cheerful.

The Surgical Team

At least four people will be present during your surgery. The *anesthesiologist*, whom you've already met and talked with, or a *registered nurse anesthesist* will put you to sleep and will continuously monitor your vital signs—heart rate, respiration, and blood pressure—during the surgery. Your temperature will also be taken at regular intervals. The anesthesiologist continues to give and monitor the anesthesia throughout your surgery and will administer any necessary fluids to maintain your circulation.

The *surgeon* performs the actual surgery and may have an assistant. If you are in a teaching hospital, residents or medical students may be present as observers. Unless there's some special circumstance, your family doctor and your medical oncologist will not be there.

The third member of the surgical team is the *circulating nurse*, who keeps track of everything that is happening. This is a big responsibility. He or she records all fluids entering and leaving your body, inventories the surgical equipment and sponges, keeps thorough charts on your progress, and also does such things as answer the phone or take care of other operating-room details.

The final member of the team is a *registered nurse* or

surgical technician, who is responsible for handing the surgeon the operating instruments as they are asked for.

Going to Sleep for Surgery

When you are brought into the surgical suite, the nurse will help you move from the gurney to the operating table. Your anesthesiologist will be there to talk to you and to tell you what's happening. Anesthesiology is such an advanced art these days that you don't need to fear what's happening, even if you have another health problem, such as a heart condition.

The anesthesiologist may tell you that you're now being given medication through your IV and might ask you to start counting. Chances are you will be asleep before you can count to ten. It's also possible that an oxygen mask will be put on your face during this time.

As you are falling asleep the operating room will seem like a very busy place, with lots of movement around you as the staff prepares to start surgery.

Once you are asleep, you will have a breathing tube put down your throat to keep your airways open. You will also have a catheter inserted in your bladder to carry off accumulating urine. The IV that was inserted earlier stays in your arm the entire time. Your breast and underarm will be cleaned. Your body will be draped with sterile sheets with only the surgical area itself exposed.

After Surgery

The amount of time you are in the surgical suite depends on what type of surgery you have. Typically, breast cancer surgery takes two to four hours. Lumpectomy patients with small tumors may be in surgery less than two hours.

When the surgeon finishes the surgery itself and is closing the incision, the anesthesiologist begins the process of waking you up by discontinuing the anesthesia. Once you are breathing on your own, the breathing tube in your throat will be removed. You may still be given oxygen.

When surgery is finished, you will be moved back to the gurney and taken to the recovery room, where you will spend the next thirty to sixty minutes waking up. The IV will still be in your arm and the urinary catheter will be in your bladder. If you had a mastectomy, you will also have one drain under your arm and one on your chest wall. If you had a lumpectomy, you will probably only have a drain under your arm. Your chest area will be swathed in a dressing of white bandages.

The Recovery Room

As you gradually become aware of your surroundings in the recovery room you will realize that a nurse is occasionally checking your pulse, respiration, and blood pressure (vital signs). She will also talk to you and ask you your name. You will probably feel drowsy and you may keep falling back asleep.

You may feel like you are coming up out of deep water, and you may or may not be in control of what you are saying. The recovery room can take on a surreal quality. As you awaken, you may notice other patients. Some will be sleeping, others will be mumbling or trying to sit up.

*　　　*　　　*

The Aftereffects of Anesthesia

You may feel cold and shiver. You may also may feel thirsty, but because the muscles in your intestines won't be working normally until the anesthesia wears off, you will not be allowed to have anything to eat or drink. Consequently, if you ask for a drink, you will probably be given only crushed ice or lemon wedges for a while.

All of these symptoms gradually go away. As soon as you can say your name to a nurse or can count the number of fingers being held before you, and when all of your vital signs are stable, you will be taken via gurney to your hospital room. The bladder catheter may be removed before you leave recovery. The IV is usually removed sometime later.

In Your Hospital Room

Friends or family members who have waited during your surgery may see you when you come out of the recovery room or will be waiting for you in your room. The nurse will continue to check you frequently once you are put into your hospital bed. She or he will monitor your vital signs and make sure you are comfortable. As soon as the urinary catheter is removed, the nurse will also encourage you to urinate frequently.

Lumpectomy Patients

Some lumpectomy patients receive a booster dose of radiation to the immediate breast area that had surrounded the tumor. This area is often referred to as the tumor bed. In some hospitals, the booster dose of radiation is given shortly after surgery via radioactive seeds loaded into tubes (catheters) implanted into the tumor bed area at the time of lumpectomy.

If you have had a lumpectomy and if you will be receiving radiation to the tumor bed via irridium implants put in place during surgery, you may have a CAT scan to check on placement of the catheters after surgery.

Visitors will be limited and will need to remain at least fifteen feet from you. A radiation oncologist will insert the irridium into the tubes once you are in your room. The radiation oncologist will continue to monitor the implants until they are removed.

While you are receiving radiation through the implants, you will have a private room and will need to stay in the room the entire time the irridium is in place. This is typically one to three days. Refer to Chapter Eight for a more detailed explanation.

Because you'll be spending a lot of time by yourself, you may want to bring a book or magazines with you. You'll be able to resume normal eating patterns fairly quickly. Once radiation treatments are completed, the seeds and catheters will be removed and you'll be able to go home.

Mastectomy Patients

If you have a mastectomy, you will be in a private or semiprivate room. It may take you longer to recover from the anesthesia than if you had a lumpectomy because you were under its effects longer.

For the first twenty-four hours or so, nurses will

monitor your vital signs every four hours. They will check the drainage from your surgical incision site and the dressing on your chest. But it will probably be your surgeon, rather than the nurses, who will change this dressing, at least the first time.

The nurses will help you to get up and to move around until you can do it on your own. They will encourage you to move the arm of the breast operated on and to start using the arm to eat or to perform tasks that do not require a lot of movement or effort. The nurses will also help you elevate the arm to prevent swelling.

Mastectomy patients usually stay in the hospital four to five days. Your insurance policy may affect the length of your stay. If at all possible, it's helpful to stay until you are self-sufficient and can bathe and take care of yourself without assistance. Because you will still have drains in your incisions, the nurses will teach you how to take care of them as well as your dressing.

Physical Pain

If you've had major surgery before, you know that for the first twenty-four hours after the surgery itself you're still pretty groggy. You may not have much discomfort the first few hours or even the first day.

In spite of your relief that the surgery is over and that the cancer has been removed, you will usually experience some physical pain once the grogginess wears off. This is because skin and underlying tissues have been cut, bruised, and stretched. Some people experience headaches after having general anesthesia. Others feel sick to their stomachs or are constipated. Pain medications, antinausea medications, and stool softeners will help. You shouldn't worry about getting addicted to them. You need to start taking them on a regular basis as soon as the problem starts instead of waiting until you are in severe pain, vomiting, or are so severely constipated that you need an enema. When you have recovered completely, you can wean yourself from these medications.

Phantom Pain in the Missing Breast

An interesting phenomenon that some women experience after a mastectomy is "phantom pain" in the area of the missing breast. These sensations may take the form of numbness, tingling, or actual stabbing pains, and are probably due to nerve endings that were cut during surgery. People who lose an arm or leg to amputation report the same sensation. Again, pain medication can help you through this difficult period.

Let Medical Personnel Know How You Feel

Fortunately, the worst physical pain will be behind you in a few days. Right after surgery, if you have no nausea or vomiting and your bowels are working, you will probably be able to drink some juice and eat soft foods, and you will rapidly start to feel better. Don't suffer in silence—tell your doctor and the medical staff how you are feeling and they will try to help you.

For some women, anxiety and depression in the immediate postoperative period are far worse than physical pain.

It may be hard for you to predict how you'll react. It may be only after surgery that you have time to think about what all this means to you. The period of time

83

between biopsy and surgery is often brief, and you may have been overwhelmed during that time with such decisions as what kind of surgery to have, where to have it, and which surgeon to have perform it.

Then you have the surgery—and boom! You're lying in a hospital bed, you touch your bandages, and the truth hits: you've had a lumpectomy or a mastectomy and part or all of your breast is gone. In addition, you may be one of the women who wonders whether all the cancer cells have been removed from your body.

The Battle Is On

This is when some women begin a psychological battle that is just as difficult as the physical battle. You need your loved ones with you now—your husband or lover, friends, and family members—those people who will give you their support and their acceptance no matter what.

Oncology nurses who work with breast cancer patients can't predict how individual women will react. Amy Strauss Tranin, oncology resource coordinator at the University of Kansas Cancer Center in Kansas City, Kansas, says that people usually cope in whatever ways they have in the past.

"Most people have been tested sometime in their lives," says Ms. Tranin, who is an R.N. "To feel anger, to want to deny what's happening, to ask over and over 'why me? why me?' is all very normal. Women who are talkers usually talk about their feelings, and women who have difficulty sharing their feelings will often try to work through it alone.

"We find the best way for our patients to cope is to talk about their feelings. The nurses will listen. After all, even if we haven't had breast cancer, we're women, and therefore we're all at risk. And we work all the time with women with breast cancer, and have been exposed to their emotions—which are very justifiable—many times."

Ms. Tranin says that some women who have mastectomies have few problems accepting what has happened to them and they only want to get well. These women usually don't flinch the first time the surgeon takes off their bandages and they see what they now look like.

Women who have mastectomies typically report that working up the courage to look at the incision is worse than actually seeing it. Like any new incision, it's going to be red and angry looking. The chest wall itself is going to be flat. The breast and the nipple are gone.

Include Your Husband in What's Happening

If you have lost a breast, confronting your new self can be traumatic. Husbands are frequently left out of this experience. They should be there to lend support so they, too, can confront this new reality. Even if you're going to go through breast reconstruction and may have started the process during your surgery, it will still be some time before reconstruction is finished and the wound is healed. In the meantime, you must come to terms with what you look like now.

And so must your husband, so have him with you. If you aren't married, try to have a loved one or a close friend with you to give you emotional support when the bandages come off.

It can also be helpful to have your advocate with you —that person you can count on to get all the information for you—because the surgeon and the nurses will be giving you information on how to take care of the incision and the drainage tubes.

Naturally you will worry about how your husband or lover will react to seeing your incision. Studies reveal that the majority do not have a negative reaction. They are far more concerned about your health than about the missing breast.

In addition to dealing with the missing breast, waiting for pathology test results is also a source of stress during the hospital stay. Typically it takes three days to get reports back, and during that time you will probably worry about what they will say and what that will mean in terms of other treatment that might be necessary.

Many women worry that they won't have the strength to resume care of children and to return to jobs when they are released from the hospital. Women with small children express the most concern.

Battling Depression

Even with good support, coming to terms with breast cancer is essentially a personal battle. When you are alone, you may find yourself feeling sad or depressed. This is normal. Don't apologize for it.

If you had a mastectomy, you are also grieving for a lost body part—a part very tied up in your feelings about your femaleness. And you are confronting your own mortality, for you can't have breast cancer and not think about the fact that some women don't survive it.

Life is an emotional land mine for you right now. You need rest, you need support from your loved ones, and you need time to adjust to what is happening to you.

Let Other People Help You

Do not be afraid to ask for help or support. When a friend or family member asks if you need anything, let them do something for you. That makes them feel good and helps you at the same time. People care and want to help. Let them!

Some women find it helpful to talk to another woman who has gone through the experience of having a mastectomy. With your doctor's permission, a volunteer from the American Cancer Society's Reach to Recovery program will come to the hospital or to your home to visit you. She has had a mastectomy and will talk to you about your concerns, give you information about exercises that will help you regain your strength (you'll read more about this in the following chapters), and leave you with a soft breast form to wear if you wish during initial recovery until you can be fitted with a prosthesis or undergo reconstruction. You are in no way obligated to the American Cancer Society to give money or to become a volunteer for them.

You may also find visits from friends, your minister, and family members to be helpful. If you don't want visitors, or if you want to specify which visitors you'd like to see, be sure to make this known to the hospital staff.

If You Go Home Before You Feel Up to It

Because many insurance companies insist that patients leave the hospital so quickly these days, you may find yourself going home before you feel up to it.

By all means, accept any help you're offered. If you

have young children at home, someone else is going to need to take care of them until you've regained your strength and the use of your arm. Until you're feeling back to normal, your number-one priority must be *you*.

Questions to Ask Your Doctor

Going into the hospital for major surgery can be a traumatic experience for anyone. The more you know, the more in control you will feel. Be sure to ask your doctor and the nurses all the questions you want answered. Don't feel that the "best" patient is the silent one. Most medical personnel are happy to tell you what you want to know and will be very helpful. As we've suggested before, you may want to write down your questions and the answers they give you so you don't forget. Remember to keep a paper and pen with you.

And remember that there is no need for you to suffer needless anxiety and pain. Let your doctor or the medical staff know when you are afraid or when you hurt. They can lend you emotional support and often have effective medications that will assist as well.

- When will I check into the hospital?
- How long will I be in the hospital?
- Are there any complications I might experience?
- How soon after surgery will I see my surgeon?
- When will my bandages be removed?
- Will I be visited by a Reach to Recovery volunteer?
- How long will it be before I can resume my normal activities?
- When will I know my pathology test results and

talk to someone about what further treatment, if any, is needed?

If you are having lumpectomy and radiation, you will find more information on what will happen to you in the hospital in the upcoming chapter on radiation.

6 When You Choose Breast Reconstruction

Today, breast reconstruction is an option for most women who have had mastectomies. This wasn't always the case. For a long time, the prevailing opinion of the medical community was that reconstruction was unnecessary surgery. Whether they meant to or not, doctors often conveyed the message to their patients that women who wanted reconstruction were vain and frivolous. They would warn them that results might not be satisfactory, and that reconstruction was painful, time-consuming, and expensive.

*   *   *

Positive Benefits of Reconstruction

Today more and more doctors are recognizing that being able to look "complete," whether dressed or undressed, can have a positive psychological impact upon a woman. Having two breasts is a part of her sense of femininity and attractiveness. No woman should have to apologize for feeling that reconstruction is important. Reestablishing feminine identity is a significant benefit of reconstruction. There are others as well.

The loss of a breast often results in a weight imbalance, which can cause neck and upper-back pain. Reconstruction can prevent this.

Reconstruction allows a woman to again be able to wear all types of clothing, including swimsuits and revealing necklines. She will also be able to participate in physical activities, such as swimming or tennis, that might be restricted or be uncomfortable if she wears a prosthesis (breast form).

Historical Developments in Breast Reconstruction

Procedures for creating a new breast for a woman who has had a mastectomy date back to before the turn of the century. The early operations pioneered techniques for transferring folds of skin and underlying tissues from other parts of the body to the chest wall to create a breast mound. Numerous surgical procedures were sometimes required, and the results could be far from satisfactory.

Injecting substances under the skin to simulate

breasts was also tried. Paraffin wax, various types of sponges, and even glass balls were used. Infections and scarring was commonplace following these types of procedures.

In the 1940s, plastic surgeons experimented with the transfer of fat and tissue from the buttocks into the breast area. They quickly learned that the body reabsorbs fat, and the only thing that remained after several years were the scars a woman now had on her bottom.

Early Silicone

One of the most disastrous attempts came in the 1960s when liquid silicone was injected under the skin of the breast area. In several documented cases, the silicone escaped the breast area and traveled into the lungs. In more than one instance, it was fatal.

The 1970s and 1980s were important decades in the progress of breast reconstruction for several reasons.

First, surgeons learned that less radical surgery than the Halsted method was just as effective in treating breast cancer, and that the extra skin and soft tissue available made reconstruction easier.

Second, implants that had a fairly natural look and feel were developed and these were far safer than previous implants.

Third, surgeons discovered that implants could be placed under the skin left by a mastectomy without interfering with the blood supply to the skin.

Finally, plastic surgeons developed a new procedure whereby skin and muscle from another part of the body —usually the back or abdomen—could be used to rebuild a breast, even if the patient had had prior radiation or a radical mastectomy.

Three Options Worth Considering

While a number of types of breast reconstruction methods are currently in use, many doctors feel the following three are the safest and give the best cosmetic results. (See Illustration #7.)

The first two involve use of implants. Reconstruction may be started (a) at the time of mastectomy, or (b) anytime thereafter, provided enough chest wall skin is available and the patient is not receiving an aggressive chemotherapy regimen.

Immediate Restoration at Time of Mastectomy

Women with very early stage breast cancer (carcinoma in situ or Stage I) can often consider starting reconstruction at the same time they have a mastectomy. They select a plastic surgeon and discuss all particulars ahead of time. The advantage is obvious: They only go through major surgery one time, and they awaken from anesthesia knowing they will still have two breasts.

This procedure is usually recommended only for very early stage breast cancer because it carries a higher risk of immediate and/or delayed infection than does mastectomy alone. Women with Stage II or III breast cancer often undergo chemotherapy, which increases the possibility of infection around the implanted prosthesis. If the prosthesis becomes infected, it usually must be removed.

During the first part of the operation, a general surgeon removes all of the breast tissue and all or most of

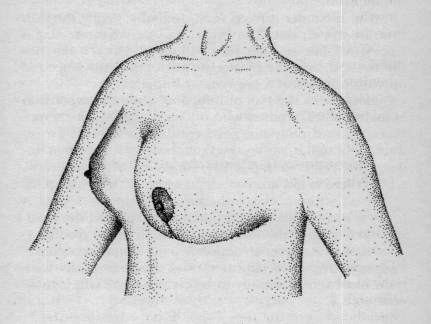

illustration 7: When all conditions are right and the plastic surgeon is skilled, breast and nipple reconstruction can yield impressive results.

the lymph nodes. The plastic surgeon then inserts a semisolid form under the chest wall muscles. This "expander" is like an empty plastic bag. Over the next several weeks, small amounts of saline solution are injected into the expander through a tube that protrudes through the incision.

The expander is filled very gradually, giving the skin time to stretch out. The breast can be whatever size a woman wishes and her skin will allow. Once it reaches the desired size, the plastic surgeon performs a second operation to insert a permanent implant.

Because of the risk of infection while the expansion is taking place, women who undergo aggressive chemotherapy are usually not good candidates for this procedure, although it has worked successfully for women undergoing mild to moderate forms of chemotherapy, where there is not a severe depression of the white cells.

Even without chemotherapy, infection is a risk. A foreign body being placed under the skin and the gradual stretching of the tissue and skin all invite trouble.

Immediate reconstruction is a fairly new procedure, and women considering it should check carefully with their insurance company to be certain costs will be covered.

Delayed Implant Reconstruction

Some women want to adjust first to the fact that they have cancer and see how they feel about reconstruction before they make the decision to have it. That's one reason for delaying reconstruction.

Also, women who need aggressive chemotherapy or who have other health problems or who must stabilize their weight or stop smoking first (smoking can cause tissue complications in breast reconstruction) are usually advised to wait. Delayed reconstruction can begin anywhere from six months after surgery to many years later.

The plastic surgeon opens the scar and puts in a tissue expander that looks something like a hot-water-bottle bladder. It creates a pocket between the muscle and bones of the chest wall. Over the next two to three months, the woman visits her doctor weekly to have small amounts of sterile fluid injected into the bladder, which gradually stretches the skin. When the correct size is attained, the plastic surgeon removes the bladder and inserts the permanent implant.

Pros and Cons of Implant Surgery

One of the advantages of implant surgery is that women who are unhappy with the size of their breasts can select the size they want during reconstruction and the remaining breast can be surgically altered to match it.

With implants, the resulting breast looks and feels fairly "natural," although it cannot have the sensations of a normal breast. Some women describe it as feeling "numb," while others claim that over the years they begin to develop feelings in the reconstructed breast.

Though most women are very pleased with the results of silicone implants, once in a while complications do arise. The body will attempt to reject any foreign substance placed in it, and if this happens, there may be inflammation around the implant or scar tissue may develop that can cause the implant to move out of place. Plastic surgeons can't predict these complications. When they occur, the implants must be removed or repositioned.

The presence of implants does increase the difficulty in X-raying the breasts if there is still breast tissue. However, this is not a problem in women undergoing reconstruction following mastectomy because the breast tissue has been removed. It's also important that women with implants be especially conscientious about breast self-examination.

In spite of concerns to the contrary, there is no data to support the fear that implants may cause a new cancer to develop in the breast.

Tissue Transfer

Tissue transfer, called the TRAM flap procedure, requires no implant. Instead, a new breast mound is formed from tissue taken from a woman's own body—generally the abdomen, the back, or the buttocks. While the forerunner of this procedure was unsuccessful when it was used in the 1940s, recent surgical advancements have improved the results.

Rectus Abdominus Reconstruction

Plastic surgeons often recommend using tissue from the abdomen for breast reconstruction because of the favorable match of skin color and texture.

During the operation, tissue is cut free from the abdomen just below the belly button to form a "flap" of muscle, skin, and fat. This flap is still connected to its artery and vein and is moved under the skin to the site of the mastectomy, formed into the shape of the breast, and sewn in place. Circulation is already established because the artery and vein are still attached, and healing proceeds quickly.

The drawback to this procedure is that loss of muscle in the abdomen can cause back pain in some women. One plus is that it in effect provides the woman with a "tummy tuck."

Latissimus Dorsi Reconstruction

When too little tissue may be left at the site of the mastectomy to hold and cover an implant, plastic surgeons sometimes recommend reconstruction using skin and muscle from the back. They create a new muscle on the front of the chest from the latissimus dorsi muscle on the back, which is located below the shoulder blade.

Once again the flap is tunneled under the skin. The blood vessels are kept intact, minimizing circulation complications, and an implant can be put behind the flap to create a larger breast.

Gluteus Free Flap

In this third procedure, the flap comes from the buttocks. Because it can't be tunneled under the skin, the vessels must be cut and reconnected to an artery and vein in the chest wall.

Pros and Cons of Flap Surgery

Flap surgery is major surgery, requiring general anesthesia and a stay in the hospital. You also run a risk of complications, such as bleeding and infection or reaction to the anesthesia. All three types of flap surgery leave scars elsewhere on the body as well. As with any kind of surgery, complications often can't be predicted.

None of these surgeries can restore sensation in the breast. That is gone forever. Women sometimes have unreal expectations of what the reconstructed breast will look or feel like. You will have scars and you will not have a completely normal breast.

As surgical procedures continue to improve, results of breast reconstruction will get better and better.

Who Is a Poor Candidate for Breast Reconstruction?

If you must have external beam radiation, you may not be a good candidate for breast reconstruction because of damage to your skin. Poor skin tone and lack of skin elasticity can also be a problem in elderly women, and in women who are diabetic or who are heavy smokers.

Even if your skin tone is passable, you may not be pleased with the overall cosmetic effects of your reconstruction. This is something that should be discussed with your plastic surgeon. You must have realistic expectations so you don't undergo this surgery only to be disappointed with the results.

Reconstructing a New Nipple and Areola

Creating a new nipple and areola (surrounding area) is another procedure that has come a long way in recent years.

Plastic surgeons graft skin from another part of the body—the upper inner thigh, from behind the ear, from the opposite nipple, or from the vaginal lips—creating the new structures. If they aren't dark enough, several procedures can be used to change the color. The new nipple will not have the usual sensation, but will make the new breast look as close to normal as possible.

Reconstruction and a Sense of Wholeness

Only you can decide if breast reconstruction is right for you. How you will react to losing one or both breasts is something even you may not be able to predict.

Some women know absolutely that they want to have breast reconstruction. Others come to this conclusion several years after their mastectomies. And others consider a missing breast a minor inconvenience and have no desire to go through more surgery or to have an artificial breast.

As we said, this is a personal decision. What's important is that *you* make it and not be embarrassed about telling your doctor you're interested in it. After all, had you lost a leg instead of a breast, you would want to talk about getting an artificial leg, wouldn't you?

Until you had your surgery, you had two breasts. They were a component of your femininity and sense of attractiveness. Some women feel they are no longer sexually attractive if they lose a breast, and on that basis alone opt for reconstruction. Others report that neither they nor their husband is bothered by the missing breast, but they wish reconstruction so that there is an equal weight on each side of their chest wall and so that their clothing will fit properly.

Talk to Other Women

If you truly can't decide what to do, members of your medical team, your primary-care physician, nurses who cared for you at the hospital, or friends and relatives may know women who have had breast cancer and have faced the same dilemma. Talking to them may help you decide what to do.

Or you may find visiting with a volunteer from the American Cancer Society will offer some valuable insight.

Remember, you don't have to make this decision immediately. If the answer isn't clear to you, you may be happiest getting through your surgery, regaining your health, and then deciding if reconstruction is important enough to you to go through with it.

Above all, make the decision for yourself. Of course you care how your husband or lover feels, but it's your body, and the decision should be yours.

Select a Qualified Plastic Surgeon

If you decide you want to have reconstruction, your next task is to select the best plastic surgeon you can find. Once again, ask for recommendations from other doctors you come in contact with and from nurses. You need more than a plastic surgeon—you need a plastic surgeon who specializes in breast reconstruction.

When you visit a plastic surgeon to discuss breast reconstruction, ask to see "before" and "after" pictures. You probably won't enjoy seeing the "before" photos, but it's very important that you do. What you are going to ask them to do is very important, and *you need to know the work they are capable of doing.*

A truly qualified plastic surgeon will willingly show you photos and will explain to you why some of the "after" photos might not be as good as he or she would have preferred.

Be sure you ask to see photos of women who are similar to you in age, breast size, and skin elasticity. It's also preferable if they are of the same race.

As with any doctor, it's important that you feel you can trust the plastic surgeon and that this person has your best interests at heart. If you feel any hesitation, try to talk to at least one other plastic surgeon who specializes in breast reconstruction before you make your decision.

Once you find a plastic surgeon you like, you can proceed to discuss which type of breast reconstruction will be best for you.

What Will Breast Reconstruction Cost?

Many factors determine the answer to this. Check your insurance coverage carefully so you know what will be paid. The plastic surgeon and the accounting department at the hospital will be able to closely estimate their costs in the event that you need this information.

Even if you have to pay for this surgery with no help from your insurance company (though most policies will cover at least a portion of it), weigh carefully what breast construction will mean to your well-being. If you decide that it is important, then its value will more than offset the cost.

*   *   *

Questions to Ask Your Doctors

- Will the planned treatment for my cancer allow me to have breast reconstruction?
- When is the best time for me to have it?
- Which type of breast reconstruction would you recommend—and why?
- How will the surgery be performed?
- What are the risks?
- How long will I be in the hospital?
- How long will the healing take?
- What will my scars look like?
- How much does this surgery cost?
- How much of this will my insurance cover?

7 Opting for a Prosthesis

When you learn you have breast cancer and will have a mastectomy, deciding whether or not to have reconstructive surgery may be one decision too many. Fortunately, this is one of very few that you don't have to make right away.

You have the option of beginning reconstruction at the time of surgery, of delaying it until you are fully healed or have more time to make your decision, or of never having it done.

Chances are, you'll at least try on a prosthesis (breast form), possibly while you're still in the hospital. This will help you to decide how you feel about it.

*   *   *

Why Some Women Decide Against Breast Reconstruction

Whether or not to have breast reconstruction should be a purely personal decision. Here are some reasons you may decide against it:

- You don't want to endure any more surgery if you can avoid it, and since this is an elective process, you want no part of it.
- You fear the results of reconstructive surgery might not be to your liking.
- Your doctor tells you that you aren't a good candidate for reconstructive surgery.
- You have no problem accepting your postsurgery body image and feel no less sexually desirable for having lost one or both breasts.
- Your husband or lover is supportive of your decision not to have reconstruction, and the two of you still find lovemaking satisfactory.

The Advantages of Wearing a Prosthesis

If you decide not to have reconstruction or learn that you're not a good candidate for it, you have the option of wearing a prosthesis. This will allow you to feel more normal because when you're dressed you look normal. You will also find that specialty stores carry lines of attractive swimwear and sportswear with a built-in prosthesis that will allow you to resume activities you might have enjoyed prior to your surgery.

Most women find wearing a prosthesis quite comfortable. Of course nothing is as good as having your own breast was, but you knew that would be the case. It's important that you invest in a good prosthesis fitted specifically for you, or you won't be happy with it at all. When a prosthesis is fitted correctly, it is not only comfortable, but under clothing it looks natural.

You may be surprised at the cost, because it can run into several hundred dollars. However, many insurance companies will pay for the prosthesis. Medicare, for example, will pay 80 percent of the cost of a prosthesis and two special bras yearly.

You won't be able to wear a breast form (prosthesis) until your chest wall is completely healed.

Acquiring a Prosthesis

Breast forms are usually filled with a liquid or gel form of silicone so that they look, feel, and have the weight of a natural breast. Shapes vary in order to give you a natural contour whether you've had radical, modified, or simple mastectomy.

Lighter forms, made of cotton or foam, are available to wear at night.

Once you know specifically what kind of breast form works best for you, you may be able to order forms through specialty catalogs. But in the beginning, you should consider being fitted by a professional who can help you select the right kind for you and can make sure it fits you properly.

Check the Yellow Pages of your phone book under "brassières" or "lingerie." Often the bra departments of major department stores have a salesperson with special training in fitting. Also, the local chapter of the American Cancer Society, a volunteer from Reach to Recovery, or the personnel in your doctor's office may be able to provide you with a list of specialty stores.

Don't be embarrassed when it's time for your fitting. The women who provide this service are sensitive to your feelings. Many of them have also had mastectomies. They will know how to measure you properly and will provide you with instructions on how to care for your breast forms.

To Wear or Not to Wear a Prosthesis

You may decide you don't want to wear anything. There is one disadvantage if you've lost just one breast, which is that your body will be off balance. You run the risk of developing problems caused by one shoulder dropping down and inward while the other is up. You are also susceptible to back, shoulder, and neck problems caused by the imbalance.

Also, if you've lost just one breast, you may experience difficulty finding clothing that will fit well on you. This is a problem you can work around, of course. And a skilled physical therapist may be able to help you develop an exercise program that will counteract the physical problems associated with having only one breast and not wearing a prosthesis on the other side.

A Different Kind of Prosthesis

Within the last several years, another option has been available to women who have had mastectomies. This is a custom-made breast prosthesis that actually adheres to the body and exactly matches the natural breast in size, shape, color, and weight.

Referred to as an "Image," because it is manufactured by a company in Pennsylvania called External Reconstruction Technology (see the referrals at the end of the book for more information), this new prosthesis is rapidly gaining acceptance among the medical community and among women who have had mastectomies.

Each Image prosthesis is custom-made. A company representative calls on a woman and explains the process. If she's interested and has no skin allergy to the substances used, she makes an appointment to have a lightweight cast made of her upper torso. This takes about thirty minutes. It's shipped to the manufacturing plant where the prosthesis is created, usually within four to six weeks. The company representative then teaches the woman how to apply it and how to care for it.

The Image can be worn for days, or even weeks at a time. It can be worn unadhered in a bra, adhered for short periods using an adhesive that washes off, or firmly anchored with a special adhesive that will allow it to remain in place for an extended period of time.

The back of the prosthesis is custom-fitted to the chest wall, while the front mirrors the natural breast. Made of silicone, it has a very lifelike appearance.

The realistic appearance of the Image prosthesis makes it a satisfactory choice for the woman who is not a good candidate for reconstruction. Most insurance companies will cover at least 80 percent of the cost.

It's Up to You

Reconstruction, prosthesis, or nothing—the choice is yours. Think carefully about each option and how it will affect your life.

And if you're unsure, you may want to start by wearing a traditional prosthesis. Perhaps after a while you'll want to try the new type of adhering prosthesis. You will have the option, even years later, to have reconstruction.

8 Radiation Therapy

Some people, when they hear the term "radiation," can only think of what happened to the victims of the atomic bomb dropped on Hiroshima in World War II. In their minds they envision people with scalded-looking skin, parched tongues, and hair that is falling out in clumps.

In truth, administration of radiation as a form of cancer treatment is very different from such a nightmare image. Handled by experienced radiation oncologists using state-of-the-art radiation equipment, it is a lifesaving therapy with limited side effects.

After surgery, women who have lumpectomies receive radiation therapy to the whole breast, the axillary node area, and sometimes to other regional node areas as well.

Sometimes women who have mastectomies also receive radiation therapy. This occurs when the risk of local (chest wall or under the arm) recurrence is high because either a large number of lymph nodes or the chest wall muscles have been invaded by the breast cancer.

Radiation therapy after lumpectomy may consist of only external beam (radiation delivered from outside the body by a machine aimed at the tumor bed) or external beam plus irridium implants (radiation delivered directly to the tumor bed without going through the outer layers of skin).

Radiation following mastectomy usually consists only of external beam treatments.

A combination of different types of external beam treatments may be used to decrease side effects.

Assistance in Saving the Breast

Radiation therapy has made it possible for many women with early-stage breast cancer to keep their breasts if they are candidates for lumpectomies (see Chapter Four on treatment options for specific information).

Like chemotherapy, radiation kills cancer cells. But it can only do so in those areas where the radiation beam is aimed. Radiation given to the whole body in a dose high enough to kill breast cancer cells would cause unacceptable toxicity or even death. The primary use of radiation in early breast cancer is to help rid the rest of the breast and skin and lymph nodes of any cancer cells remaining in the local area after the lumpectomy.

Chemotherapy, on the other hand, is a whole-body (systemic) treatment that goes after any cancer cells that may have escaped to other parts of the body.

The advantage of radiation is that damage to healthy cells occurs mainly in the radiated area, while chemotherapy may affect healthy cells throughout the body.

The Development of Radiation Therapy

In 1898 when Madame Marie Curie discovered radium, the first radioactive element discovered, she recognized its effect on human cells and envisioned using it to treat cancer patients.

It wasn't until 1924 that breast cancer patients were first treated with radiation therapy. Through the years, researchers have learned about correct dosages to administer and how to target the radiation beams in order to cause as little damage as possible to surrounding tissue. Radiation equipment has evolved from low-dose instruments that left most of the radiation in the skin, to powerful high-energy electron beams that take the radiation to specified depths in specified areas.

In addition, researchers and radiologists have learned how to administer radiation internally, taking it directly to the source of the tumor without going through external layers of skin and tissue.

Some women receive both types of radiation. Deciding how and when to administer radiation therapy involves many factors, including a woman's overall health, her age, and to some extent, her preferences and those of her doctor.

Treatment itself is painless, but the experience can be traumatic if you don't know what to expect.

*   *   *

Radiation Implants After Lumpectomy

Following lumpectomy, most patients receive radiation to the whole breast and axillary nodes. Many radiation oncologists also boost (radiate) the small area called the tumor bed (where the tumor was found) with an even higher dose of radiation. This is thought to give even greater protection against tumor recurrence.

Some radiation oncologists perform the entire treatment with external beam radiation using a powerful machine positioned above the patient. Others use irridium implants for the boost, feeling they provide better protection and a better cosmetic result.

The irridium implants are usually put in place in the breast at the time of the axillary dissection and re-excision of the lumpectomy site while the patient is under general anesthesia.

In simplest terms, the surgeon implants a grouping of hollow plastic tubes in the breast at the site of the previous tumor. The tubes look like little straws or skewers with screw-on caps on the ends. How many are implanted—from ten to twenty or so—depends on the size of the tumor. (See Illustration #8.)

If the low-dose delivery method is used, approximately twenty-four hours later the irridium is loaded into the tubes, where it remains for twenty to sixty hours. Then the tubes are removed.

Required Isolation

If you have low-dose radiation implants, you will need to remain in a hospital room in semi-isolation dur-

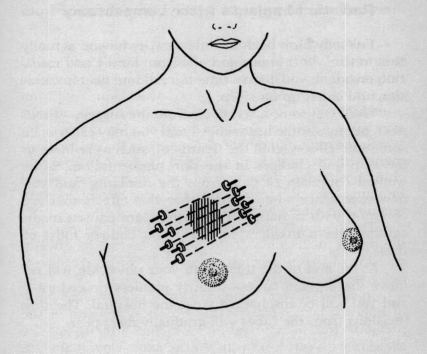

illustration 8: Under general anesthesia, radioactive seeds of irridium are added to fine plastic tubes inserted into the breast at the site of the tumor bed to destroy any remaining cancer cells. The number of tubes depends on the dosage of radiation to be used and the area to be covered.

ing the two to three days of implant treatment. Close family members may be able to visit for an hour at a time, but will be required to stay some distance from you.

You may look back on this time as having actually been restful. With minimal visits from family and medical personnel, you'll have time to read and watch television and catch up on sleep.

You'll feel some aftereffects from the surgery—tiredness, perhaps some headaches—and you may experience some side effects from the treatment, such as redness to the skin and changes in the skin pigmentation. Some women complain of pain from the implants, and you may experience some of the other side effects that are common with radiation. Fortunately, antinausea medications and painkillers can help you control most of these.

At the end of the treatment, your physician will remove the implant tubes—a fairly painless procedure—and you will be discharged from the hospital. The tiny incisions from the tubes will gradually disappear.

High-Dose Treatment

New technology now makes it possible to receive implant radiation on an outpatient basis, after the tubes are implanted during surgery. Rather than stay in the hospital, women can report to the outpatient center at their hospital and have a half-hour treatment in which they receive a highly concentrated dose of radiation.

The equipment to deliver this technology is fairly new and quite expensive, so high-dose radiation is not yet available in many places.

External Beam Radiation After Lumpectomy

If you've had a CAT scan, you know the strange feeling of being treated by a huge machine that makes unusual noises and seems very large and powerful.

The radiation equipment used in external beam radiation is like that. You will be asked to put on a hospital gown and to lie down on a table in the radiation suite. The machine above you will seem monstrous in size and can be frightening, especially the first time. (See Illustration #9.)

Several days before this you will have had X rays and some other tests to help determine the exact areas to be treated and the correct dose of radiation to use. In order to spare surrounding tissue just as much as possible, lead blocks or shields may be custom-cut for you to minimize radiation exposure everywhere except the treatment area.

The radiation oncologist (sometimes called the radiation therapist) and technicians assisting you will use a pen similar to a Magic Marker to mark on your body the places where you are to receive treatment. They will tell you that these markings need to remain there throughout your treatment and warn you not to scrub them off.

Most women report that the first treatment is the hardest because they are facing a new procedure and meeting new technicians.

It may take as long as a half hour to get you properly positioned under the radiation machine. Treatment itself only takes a minute or two. As with a mammogram or dental X ray, all medical personnel will leave the room and you will hear the machine hum (some people say it

117

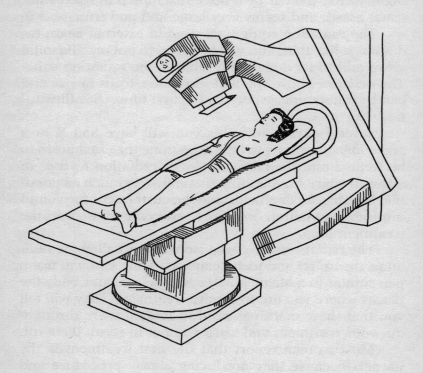

illustration 9: When a woman receives external beam radiation therapy, getting the machine properly positioned takes much longer than the treatment itself.

sounds like a vacuum cleaner) as beams of radiation pass into your body.

The Challenge of Treatment

Some women think those seconds of treatment seem like hours. They feel helpless under that huge machine and they feel very alone, even though they know technicians can see into the room and are watching them carefully.

The technicians leave the room because they do this work all day long, and radiation is very powerful. Its effects may be cumulative; constant exposure could prove harmful to them.

While radiation can be dangerous to technicians after long-term exposure, it's your friend. And it's a powerful friend, one that's capable of killing your cancer cells. If you can train yourself to relax during treatment, and if you can envision the radiation as healing rays helping to restore your good health, you'll get through the experience better than someone full of fears, who tenses up and makes the experience difficult for medical personnel as well as herself.

The Treatment Schedule

One of the advantages of external beam radiation is that most women can continue working if they wish while they are going through treatments. Appointment times can be set up early in the morning, at noon, or in the evening, to accommodate work schedules if you live near a treatment center and are able to go back to work.

Most radiation oncologists prescribe daily radiation

119

treatments, Monday through Friday, for three to six weeks, beginning as quickly as possible after surgery. This is quite a commitment of time, and it's certainly easier if you live near a good radiation center. If you don't, it may be necessary for you to take an apartment temporarily that is near the medical center or treatment center in order to receive radiation.

Such an arrangement also has the advantage of giving you adequate time to rest between treatments, because you may find yourself feeling very tired as treatment progresses.

Side Effects from Radiation Treatment

Many women suffer no adverse effects at all from radiation. Others feel constant fatigue. In the hands of a skilled radiation oncologist, cosmetic side effects will be minimal. If you are fortunate, you will notice few permanent changes in the appearance of your skin. Radiation kills whatever cells are in its path. Healthy cells will regenerate in a few weeks' time. But while you're undergoing treatment you may experience the following:

- Dry, flaky skin; itchy skin.
- Reddening and increased sensitivity of the treated skin that resembles sunburn.
- Blistering and cracking of the treated skin.
- Irritation and dryness in the throat; irritation to the esophagus.
- Nausea and vomiting.
- Alterations in taste.
- Shrinkage of breast tissue, reducing the size of the treated breast and an increase in breast skin thickness and pigmentation.

Effects on the Skin

For several weeks after you receive radiation, your skin in the radiated area will be red. This "sunburn" may be quite noticeable, but it fades with time, and the long-term effect is usually minimal. Just like a sunburn on the outer layer of the skin, it will eventually peel. If cracks or blisters appear, your treatments may be temporarily interrupted until they heal.

The treated breast may decrease in size over the next several months to years. In addition, the treated breast may feel firmer or harder than the untreated breast.

Finally, you may have increased breast skin thickness and what resembles a permanent suntan over some parts of the breast or armpit (axilla). Still, most women are satisfied with the cosmetic results after radiation.

Side effects must be balanced against the benefits of treatment, and radiation can be very effective indeed, capable of shrinking a tumor and killing cancer cells. And when it is combined with lumpectomy, the breast remains whole and it retains normal sensation and appearance.

Finding Good Treatment

External radiation and radiation implants must be administered by highly trained medical personnel. Your oncologist and surgeon can guide you in selecting a reputable, experienced radiation oncologist to direct your radiation treatment.

As with all other factors in your war against cancer,

you need to be involved in the search for the best care you can get. Breast cancer radiation therapy is a precise science, and even though a radiation oncologist may be skillful in treating other types of cancer, he or she may not be experienced in administering this very specialized treatment.

You must also consider the kind of equipment available in a hospital or treatment center. You want to be treated with state-of-the-art machinery. This may require that you drive to a medical center some distance from your home, or as we've already mentioned, you may even need to move near the medical center or cancer treatment center for a few weeks, traveling home on weekends until your radiation therapy is finished. While this can seem inconvenient and expensive, it must be weighed against the outcome.

Receiving a Combination of Radiation and Chemotherapy

If your cancer is fast growing or is large and aggressive, your medical treatment team may feel you should receive both radiation and chemotherapy. (Chemotherapy is discussed in depth in Chapter Nine.) The objective is to zap every cancer cell in your body. To accomplish this, the team will treat them at the source with radiation, then use chemotherapy to kill any cells that may have escaped to other places in your body.

There are several ways chemotherapy and radiation can be combined. You may receive chemotherapy first, then be given external radiation later. Or, you may start external beam radiation and chemotherapy at the same time. It's also possible that you may have radiation implants put in place, then be given chemotherapy, and when it's completed, have external beam radiation.

Administering both chemotherapy and radiation at the same time is tricky because it's harder on your body than either treatment alone. Both can cause your white-blood-cell count to drop, making you susceptible to infection. Both can also irritate the esophagus, making it difficult to swallow food. Some types of chemotherapy can intensify the effects of radiation on the underlying lung or heart tissue. Chemotherapy can also intensify the skin reaction caused by radiation.

Your treatment schedule may have to be modified from the one originally planned for you as medical personnel discover how well you tolerate treatment.

Radiation Recall

A problem some women encounter is called radiation recall. Chemotherapy can cause the sunburned appearance of the skin to recur, even when the skin has previously healed and chemotherapy has been given only after all radiation is completed. Usually this is a mild reaction. However, sometimes the skin can become very tender and it may peel or blister.

If you suffer from radiation recall, proper care of the skin in the affected area is very important. You'll want to do everything you can to prevent irritation or infection. You'll need to wear loose clothing and keep the affected skin out of extremes of temperature.

*   *   *

The Psychological Challenge

Your medical team will plan your treatment program very carefully, deciding when and how to combine these two therapies. Going through both of them will be a difficult time for you, not only because you must be so careful not to get sick, but also because you may feel you have no energy and no interest in eating. If you are also losing your hair or suffering from other side effects, you may find this time to be as stressful as, or even more stressful than, recovery from surgery.

Try to take it one day at a time. Don't try to work when you don't feel like it, and don't undertake any long-drawn-out projects. Instead, do as many enjoyable things as possible. Dress attractively even when you don't feel well—and you'll feel a little better.

Questions to Ask Your Doctor

- Am I a candidate for radiation therapy?
- If so, why?
- What results do you expect from it?
- What type of radiation therapy will I receive?
- Where will I have it?
- If I'm to have chemotherapy and radiation therapy at the same time, how will the schedule be worked out?
- What are the qualifications of the treatment center and of those individuals treating me?
- How long will it take?
- What side effects might I experience?

- How severe will they be and how long will they last?
- Will I be able to maintain a regular schedule of activities during my therapy?

9 Chemotherapy

As you already know, surgery and radiation are often not the end of your treatment for breast cancer. Many women proceed with adjuvant systemic therapy—which means treatment directed at the whole body that is given in addition to the therapy directed at the breast.

The purpose of adjuvant systemic therapy is to destroy any cancer cells that may have escaped the primary tumor or cancerous lymph glands before they were removed. This is done either by killing the cancerous cells with chemicals (chemotherapy), or by depriving them of the hormones they need to grow (hormone therapy) in the event tests have shown that a woman's cancerous cells contain estrogen or progesterone receptors.

Adjuvant therapy is one area of breast cancer treatment that has changed markedly in recent years because of the development of powerful new drugs and diagnostic tools, along with our increased understanding of how to destroy cancer cells.

Your medical oncologist, working with the radiation oncologist and your surgeon, will determine what adjuvant therapy you should receive. Generally, women with breast cancer fall into one of four categories: (1) they need no further treatment, or (2) they need hormone therapy, (3) chemotherapy, or (4) both hormone therapy and chemotherapy.

The category you fit into will help determine what treatment you will receive along with surgery and/or radiation.

Chemotherapy

Chemotherapy is a word that can strike fear into the hearts of breast cancer patients. They envision gaunt, bald-headed women suffering from nausea and vomiting.

In reality, many patients tolerate chemotherapy very well. They continue with careers and social activities, often without others even knowing they're going through treatment. There are many different ways to take chemotherapy drugs in order to diminish side effects. New medicines are also helping to counteract side effects.

But how a woman will physically react to a prescribed chemotherapy regimen is highly variable. True, some women barely seem to slow down during treatment, while other women are temporarily incapacitated and have such low energy levels that they can't keep up with normal activities.

A woman's chemotherapy tolerance is affected by

her basic health, her age, her natural abilities to recover, the kind of chemotherapy drugs she is being given, and how they are administered.

Many women try to squeeze chemotherapy into an already overcrowded schedule filled with demands of job and family, and some of them become ill from exhaustion.

Because the cancer-killing drugs used in chemotherapy are so powerful, going through treatment is hard on the body. While the cancer cells are succumbing to it, so, unfortunately, are healthy cells. Recognize this, and accept that you need to take very good care of yourself during this time. Healthy cells damaged by chemotherapy need time to repair themselves.

During the course of your treatment, family members may have to do more for themselves. Spouses may have to take over many chores you have always handled. Friends' offers of help should be accepted. Employers may have to be flexible. It's very possible you'll need to miss a few days of work or cut back on your work load. If you're self-employed, you may have to let your business coast for a while. Right now the most important thing is for you to regain your health, and successful chemotherapy treatments are part of that.

How Chemotherapy Works

One of the characteristics of cancer cells is that they grow erratically, and often quickly. Chemotherapy works by preventing cell division and/or by poisoning some part of the cell mechanism in order to deprive the cancer cell of the nutrients it needs to live or divide.

Some cells respond to chemotherapy, and some don't. As a general rule, cells that grow and divide rapidly (which can be determined with lab tests) respond better to chemotherapy than do cells that grow and divide slowly.

But even cells that grow and divide quickly may be resistant to chemotherapy. There are several reasons why. One is that some cells can actually "protect" themselves against certain chemotherapy drugs. Many of the body's cells have the ability to eject poisonous substances that attack them. Some chemotherapy drugs activate this type of response in the cells the drug attacks, and the cells "pump out" the drug before it can destroy them.

As a rule, the greater the number of cancer cells, the more likely that some will be resistant to the killing effects of chemotherapy. This is why chemotherapy should usually be started as soon after surgery as possible. Indeed, there are some experimental programs in which chemotherapy is started after the initial diagnostic biopsy and *before* the definitive surgery.

When Chemotherapy Isn't Indicated

Woman with noninvasive breast cancer (cancer that hasn't gotten out of the ducts and lobules into the surrounding breast tissue) do not need to have chemotherapy or hormone therapy after their surgery.

Women who have invasive breast cancer, but whose tumors are less than a half inch in size (one centimeter) and whose nodes are negative (cancer free) generally do not need chemotherapy or hormone therapy.

A woman who is node negative and whose tumor measures one-half to one-and-a-half inches (one to three centimeters) in size, and whose tumor or cancerous cells have the following characteristics, usually will not receive chemotherapy:

- Well differentiated (looks similar to normal breast tissue).
- Normal number of chromosomes.
- Low S-phase (slow growing).
- Strongly estrogen and progesterone positive.

When Chemotherapy Is Indicated

Women who have a 30 percent or greater risk of recurrence of cancer should always be considered for adjuvant, hormone, or chemotherapy. Women with positive nodes always have a 30 percent or greater chance of recurrence.

Women who have negative nodes and whose tumor is larger than one-half inch (one centimeter) in size may have a 30 percent or greater chance of recurrence and are also candidates for adjuvant treatment if their tumors exhibit one or more of the following:

- A fast-growing (S-phase measurement) tumor.
- A poorly differentiated (doesn't resemble normal breast tissue) tumor.
- Cancer cells that have invaded breast blood vessels and lymph channels.
- A tumor that is estrogen and progesterone receptor negative.
- A strong family history of breast cancer (mother, sister).
- An age of less than forty.
- Too much of the oncogenes EGFR or Her-II-neu in their cells.

The Drugs

The most commonly administered chemotherapy drugs for early breast cancer are Cytoxan, Methotrexate, Prednisone, 5-Fluorouracil (5-FU), Vinblastine, Vincristine, Adriamycin, and Mitoxantrone.

Other drugs that may be used are Cisplatin, Etoposide (VP-16), Melphalan, and Mitomycin-C.

How the Drugs Are Selected

Each of these drugs has a different way of killing cancer cells. Consequently, they are often combined in order to have the best chance of killing all the cancer cells.

Several combinations of these drugs have been shown to be effective in very advanced or metastatic breast cancer (Stage IV), causing tumors to shrink to half their original size between 50 to 70 percent of the time. When shrinkage like this happens, we say a remission has occurred.

Although remissions are common in very advanced or metastatic disease, cures are rare. This is because the tumor cells have generally been present long enough that some of them have spontaneously changed or "mutated" and have become resistant to the killing effects of the chemotherapy medicines.

In patients with earlier-stage disease (I to III), resistance to all drugs is less likely to occur. Thus, by giving adjuvant or prophylactic chemotherapy to patients with Stage I to Stage III breast cancer who are at high risk for recurrence, we have a better chance of killing all the cancer cells and getting a cure than we have by waiting until the recurrence is apparent on scans or X rays.

Clinical trials sponsored by cancer institutes of many countries have shown that prophylactic or adjuvant chemotherapy used with surgery and with or without radiation can increase the cure rate over that seen with surgery and/or radiation alone. However, chemotherapy treatment is not perfect. The further advanced the stage, the less likely the chemotherapy will completely eradicate all the cancer cells that may have escaped from the breast area. This is one of the reasons—especially for patients who have Stage II or III disease—you will be encouraged to start chemotherapy as quickly as possible after surgery.

There are many good chemotherapy combinations being used and your doctors will know what these are. But the more drugs you take, the higher your risk of side effects. Also, some combinations of drugs are more toxic than others, even though the number of drugs used is the same. The more toxic regimens are generally used in patients whose tumors have shown the most aggressive growth characteristics.

The choice of a proper drug or drugs also depends on many individual things, including the perceived aggressiveness of your cancer, your general health (which includes your heart, liver, and lung function), and your life-style.

Clinical Trials

Your oncologist may mention to you the possibility of participating in a clinical trial. Research into the causes and treatment of breast cancer is going on all over the country. Chemotherapy is an area of high activity, with many new drugs in development. Before a promising new drug or a new combination of older drugs can be marketed to the general public, tests are conducted in clinical trials on volunteers.

If you volunteer to participate in a clinical trial, you will receive standard treatment, plus something additional. That "something" will be the new treatment. Sometimes the "experimental" treatment is actually a combination of drugs given in a new manner to try to decrease side effects or to increase the cancer-killing power. Whatever it is, you will have the opportunity to benefit from it, and also to contribute to the scientific knowledge needed to further research. Keep in mind that the lifesaving treatment you are receiving now was first tested on patients in clinical trials in order to prove it effective.

The Choice Is Yours

If you have no desire to participate in experimental research or feel it would be unsafe, you have absolutely no obligation to do so. On the other hand, participating in a clinical trial may offer you the benefit of treatment not yet available to the general public.

Most oncologists are involved in national clinical trials, and they in turn involve some of their patients. About 10 percent of breast cancer patients are appropriate participants in one of the national clinical trials going on at any one time. The rest are not appropriate candidates because they don't wish to participate, because they don't fulfill the entry requirements, or because participating in the trial would not be in their best interest for reasons related to their age, work, or other health problems.

And always remember that clinical trials involve a certain amount of risk, because the treatment in the "experimental" portion of these trials can have some unknown dangers.

You will be asked to sign a consent form if you wish to participate, and at any time you can withdraw from the trial.

How Chemotherapy Is Given

Sometimes breast cancer patients have a choice of how to receive chemotherapy. There are three ways that most chemotherapy drugs are administered.

Some drugs can be given orally. The patient takes a pill or liquid that passes through the mouth and down the throat and into the bloodstream via the lining of the stomach or upper intestines.

While most patients would prefer the oral method, it won't work with some drugs because they might damage the stomach lining or not be absorbed well enough by the body.

The second way chemotherapy can be given is by using a needle to inject the drug beneath the skin or into a muscle. This allows the drug to be slowly absorbed into the bloodstream. (See Illustration #10.) Very few drugs can be given this way because many are irritating to skin and muscle.

A third method of administering chemotherapy, and the most common, is to inject it directly into the bloodstream through a vein. This can be done by injecting it rapidly into a vein or infusing the medication more slowly through an IV hookup.

The oncologist will determine which method to use by deciding how rapidly the drug should enter the blood-

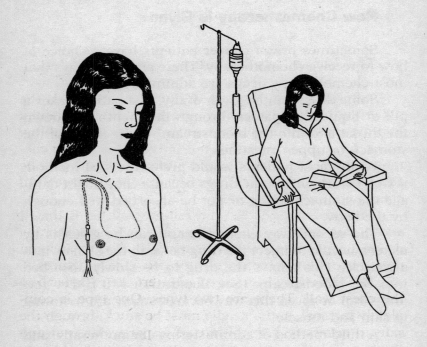

illustration 10: Chemotherapy can be administered by pill. It can also be administered via a central venous catheter that is tunneled under the chest wall skin and then empties into a major vein (illustration on the left). Or it can be administered through an IV solution that drips into a peripheral vein (illustration on the right).

stream. Rapid injection by needle often produces more side effects than does prolonged intravenous infusion. Adriamycin is one example of a chemotherapy drug that if given rapidly in large doses over long periods of time may cause damage to the heart. This risk can be lessened by giving the same drug dose over a prolonged time period (days versus minutes). Adriamycin can also cause nausea and vomiting if it's given by injection, and these side effects can also be lessened if the drug is given more slowly.

The Indwelling Catheter

Administering a drug slowly often requires that the patient have a permanent indwelling catheter implanted into the chest wall. This catheter is the size of IV tubing. Blood can usually be drawn out of the catheter and chemotherapy drugs and other nutritional products may be administered through it. The catheter stays in place until chemotherapy is completed.

The advantage of the indwelling catheter is that it allows for continuous infusion of the chemotherapy drugs directly into the bloodstream. It also means you don't have the discomfort of repeated vein punctures.

Minor surgery is required to insert the catheter into the chest wall. There are two types. One type is completely internal, and a needle must be stuck through the skin to access it. The other type is partly internal and partly external, and no skin puncture is required to access it. If the latter type of catheter is used, the soft plastic tubes dangle on the front of your chest. During the time you wear it, you will not be able to participate in some sports, swim, or submerge it in bathwater. However, you can shower, and you'll be able to do most other activities. You'll want to be careful that you do nothing that might puncture the tubes, and you'll want to wear loose-fitting clothing for comfort.

You'll receive instructions on daily care of the catheter in order to prevent infection and clotting. If you develop problems, they can usually be cleared up with medication. Only rarely must catheters be removed.

What Chemotherapy Feels Like

If you receive chemotherapy by injection, it will be like having blood drawn in a laboratory, followed by a brief cool or slight burning sensation. If you receive it by an IV infusion, you probably won't feel anything. How tense or relaxed you are when it is administered will probably affect how pleasant or unpleasant the experience is.

Some breast cancer patients administer their own chemotherapy, particularly if it's by capsule, liquid, or pill. Intravenous injections are usually administered in a clinic, doctor's office, or hospital. To some degree, how you receive chemotherapy depends on your level of tolerance, convenience, and your doctor's preferred method of treatment.

Some patients have their first chemotherapy treatments in the hospital so that the medical staff can closely monitor any side effects from the medicine. If necessary, they can change the dosage, or give additional medicines to combat any side effects. In the majority of cases, chemotherapy is administered on an outpatient basis, especially after the first dose.

Length and Frequency of Treatment

Adjuvant chemotherapy, which means chemotherapy given to kill any remaining cancer cells not detected by X ray or blood tests, usually begins shortly after surgery or after radiation treatments are completed. Sometimes it is given before radiation or it may be given after the "boost" radiation to the tumor bed, but before the external beam radiation to the whole breast. How chemotherapy will be administered, how often, and for what length of time are decisions your medical oncologist will make. These decisions, as you know, depend on many factors regarding the stage of your breast cancer, the kinds of drugs you will receive, and your emotional and physical health.

Adjuvant chemotherapy typically lasts six months to a year. During this time you may receive a particular drug daily, weekly, or monthly. Your oncologist will discuss a treatment plan with you and will also monitor it along the way, adjusting it if there is a need.

While you are undergoing chemotherapy you will need to have frequent physical examinations, scans, and medical tests to check your progress.

Side Effects

The possibility of side effects is what worries nearly every patient who undergoes chemotherapy. As we've mentioned, some women maintain their normal lifestyle, barely slowing down during chemotherapy treatments. Others suffer from vomiting, nausea, fatigue, and hair loss. Numbness or a burning sensation in the fingers and hands can also be temporary side effects, depending on the drugs used. How much a woman suffers from side effects depends on the drug or combination of drugs she is given and on her own tolerance level.

Fortunately, almost all side effects are temporary, gradually easing once chemotherapy is discontinued. Cancer researchers are actively looking for ways to reduce and control side effects.

Even if chemotherapy makes you ill and uncomfortable, taking it is very important. Remember, these powerful drugs are one of your best weapons against any cancer cells that have escaped from your breast tumor to other parts of the body. This benefit usually outweighs side effects.

Because these drugs are so powerful, they also kill healthy cells. They temporarily damage hair reproduction cells. They can lower your white-blood-cell count and put you at risk for infection, since it's the white blood cells that fight infection.

They can also decrease platelets, causing you to bruise easily, get little blood blisters under your skin, or find that it takes a long time to stop the bleeding from a cut. Most may also damage a developing baby if you should happen to get pregnant during this time. Consequently, it's very important that you take birth control precautions.

A number of these medicines can decrease the output of female hormones by the ovaries. This may cause you to have hot flashes or to stop menstruating. You may also gain weight.

It's very important that you take extremely good care of yourself during the time you are on chemotherapy. Plenty of rest, lack of stress, and good nutrition must be part of your daily life. While you may be unhappy with weight gain, *do not* try to lose weight rapidly while you are on chemotherapy.

Controlling Side Effects

Because symptoms vary from individual to individual, you will need to experiment to find out what gives you the most relief. There are a number of medications that are very helpful. The time of day you receive chemotherapy may affect you. Some women prefer to have treatment late in the day, followed by a sleeping pill so that they sleep through some of the side effects.

What you eat and when you eat it can help you control the nausea. Eat small amounts of foods. Your doctors and medical personnel will have suggestions for you.

Hair Loss

A distressful side effect is hair loss. The hair follicles contain fast-growing cells that may be affected by chemotherapy, depending on the drug. Even if the hair doesn't fall out, the scalp may get sore and the hair may become dry and lifeless. Hair loss may include all types of body hair, including the eyebrows and eyelashes.

Many women say that losing the hair on their heads is as traumatic as losing a breast—even though they know their hair will grow back. Perhaps it's because of the visibility of hair. A bald head on a woman is a sure sign of her illness.

It Helps If You Prepare Ahead of Time

If you lose your hair, it may happen gradually or within a matter of days or weeks. The best advice is to try to be prepared. Be fitted for a wig ahead of time—one that looks and feels as natural as possible and matches your natural hair color. If you can get used to wearing it ahead of time, it will be less of a shock when you actually put it on. Many insurance companies will pay for a wig if your doctor writes a prescription for it. And if you invest in a good one, few people will even realize you are wearing it.

You may also wish to invest in colorful scarves and/or hats to wear while you are going through chemotherapy. Some women find them more comfortable than a wig, and they are always an accepted fashion statement.

If you're taking fast-acting drugs that are rapidly eliminated from the body after administration once or twice a month, you may find that wearing a specially designed ice cap on your head while you're taking treatment will decrease or even prevent hair loss. But be warned: Many oncologists are uneasy about this and prefer not to do it because the scalp contains many blood vessels, and if cancer cells have already migrated there, use of an ice cap will decrease the ability of the drugs to kill those cells. And that's *not* a wise trade-off for saving some hair that will eventually grow back anyway.

Makeup Also Helps

Eyebrow pencils, eyeliner, and fake eyelashes carefully applied can lessen the shock of facial hair loss, and if you'll practice with them ahead of time, you'll be ready to use them if and when the time comes.

It's important that you maintain a sense of well-being about your looks during this time. Women sometimes become so depressed about their appearance that they refuse to go out of the house or to allow friends to visit. Such isolation only complicates the psychological problems that can accompany breast cancer.

Chemotherapy and Sterility

One other side effect that can be devastating if you're a young woman who has not yet had children is sterility. Sometimes this is temporary, and sometimes it's permanent. You must try to prepare yourself for this eventuality.

On the other hand, some drugs will not make you infertile, and you'll want to be very careful not to get pregnant while you're on chemotherapy because of complications the drugs could cause to the fetus. If you are still menstruating when you begin chemotherapy, be sure to discuss this issue with your doctor.

If your tumor is estrogen receptor positive and you have not yet gone through menopause, part of your treatment may be surgical removal of your ovaries or suppression of estrogen production of the ovaries with injections of medicines such as Zoladex.

Coming to grips with infertility may mean seeking

the assistance of a professional counselor who can help you work through your feelings.

Major Drugs and Side Effects

These are some of the major drugs currently used in breast cancer chemotherapy, and their potential side effects:

Doxorubicin
(Adriamycin)

This potent drug can cause some unpleasant side effects, including hair loss, nausea, and vomiting. Some women report that the soles of their feet and their palms and nails darken. It can also cause the urine to turn reddish in color. While the red urine is harmless and only lasts for a day or two, it can be startling.

This drug usually causes a marked decrease in the white-blood-cell count. It may decrease the platelet count as well. It can temporarily have an adverse effect on the way the heart beats. It can have a negative cumulative effect on the strength of the heart's pumping action and cause severe irritation or even death of normal tissue if it leaks out of the vein. It may also cause sores in the mouth and may exacerbate previous tissue irritation resulting from radiation.

Dihydorxyanthracenedione (DHAD)
(Mitoxantrone)

Mitoxantrone is a drug very similar to Adriamycin, but less nausea, vomiting, and heart toxicity are associated with its administration. When used as a single agent, it is not quite as active in breast cancer as Adriamycin, but it is as effective when used in combination with 5-FU and Cytoxan.

Mitoxantrone may decrease your white-blood-cell count, which can make you more vulnerable to infection. The lowering of the platelet count can make it easy for you to bruise and it may take longer for a cut to stop bleeding. These effects are temporary.

Sometimes the vein into which the drug is injected may become discolored or inflamed. Also, because of the blue color of the drug, you may find that your urine turns green for one to two days after treatment. This is harmless.

Some women experience mild nausea and/or vomiting and partial temporary hair loss.

More serious is the possibility that Mitoxantrone will affect the heart's strength, so that it can no longer pump appropriately. The more doses you receive of the drug, the greater the risk. Of lesser concern is the ability of the drug to change the way your heart beats, which may appear as electrocardiographic (EKG) changes. Generally, however, the effects of Mitoxantrone on the heart are not as severe as those caused by Adriamycin.

Cyclophosphamide
(Cytoxan)

Stomach upset is common with Cytoxan. Loss of appetite, nausea, and/or vomiting usually come on about six hours after the drug is given and last for up to four hours. Hair loss all over the body can occur, but hair will grow back when treatment ends.

Because the drug will decrease the white-cell count, you may be more vulnerable to infection. It can also lower your red-cell count, producing symptoms of shortness of breath, weakness, and fatigue. Low platelets (blood-clotting factors) can make you susceptible to bruising and bleeding for longer times. While blood problems are temporary, transfusions of red cells and platelets can counteract some of them, if needed. White-cell transfusions are not useful because of their extremely short life span.

Sometimes the bladder becomes irritated, causing pain and the appearance of blood in the urine. Drinking plenty of water (eight to ten glasses a day) and emptying your bladder frequently will help prevent this problem. Also, you should never take Cytoxan just before going to bed at night.

Once in a great while, when taken for long periods of time, Cytoxan can cause scarring of the lungs, bringing on coughing spells and shortness of breath.

Cytoxan can also cause irregular menstrual periods and temporary or permanent sterility.

Very rarely, Cytoxan has been known to actually cause a second cancer (leukemia), a risk that must be weighed against the risk of not treating your disease with this very effective drug.

Vincristine

Common side effects of this drug are constipation and stomach cramps. Stool softeners and laxatives will often prevent this. Ask your doctor. Vincristine also commonly causes numbness and tingling of the fingers and toes. This is not serious, but should the numbness progress to actual muscle weakness, the drug must be stopped. It may cause severe irritation or death of normal tissue if it leaks out of the vein.

Less common side effects include blurred or double vision, pain in various places of the body—especially the jaw, muscles, and bones, difficulty urinating, an increase in urination, and an increase in blood pressure. Very rarely the drug can cause shortness of breath, sores, and cough, fever, or chills.

It is generally not associated with severe hair loss when given by itself or with marked suppression of the white blood cells or platelets. The neurologic side effects from Vincristine can persist for months to years after the treatment is stopped.

Vinblastine

Mouth sores, loss of appetite, nausea, vomiting, diarrhea or constipation, and hair loss are side effects often experienced with this drug.

As with many other chemotherapy drugs, this one usually temporarily lowers white-cell, red-cell, and platelet counts, making you more vulnerable to infection, shortness of breath, weakness, fatigue, easier bruising, and longer bleeding time. Blood transfusions can counteract some of these symptoms, should they occur.

Some women experience headaches with this drug. In addition, Vinblastine can cause all the side effects listed for Vincristine. As with Vincristine, side effects usually disappear when drug treatment ends. However, neurologic effects of any treatment may persist for some time.

Prednisone

Side effects of Prednisone include indigestion, nervousness or restlessness, increase in appetite and weight gain, trouble sleeping, a false sense of well-being, and an increased tendency to get mouth infections and vaginal yeast infections.

Drinking alcohol may cause stomach problems if you're on Prednisone. If you're going to be on it for a long time, you may need to follow a low-salt diet and/or a potassium-rich diet. You should also take medicine to decrease the amount of acid in your stomach. If you're diabetic, Prednisone may affect your blood sugar levels.

Side effects you should report to your doctor include blurred vision, frequent urination, increased thirst, skin problems, muscle cramps, weakness, or pain, depression, menstrual problems, irregular heartbeats, black tarry stools, a rounded face, sore throat and fever, swelling of the legs or feet, excessive tiredness or weakness, and wounds that do not heal.

You may also experience some fatigue immediately after you discontinue taking Prednisone.

5-Fluorouracil

5-Fluorouracil (5-FU) can affect the gastrointestinal tract (stomach and intestine), causing loss of appetite, nausea, and/or vomiting. You may also experience mouth sores, which last a couple of days, and temporary loss of hair all over your body. It can also cause the same blood problems as the other drugs.

If you take 5-Fluorouracil, you may also notice thinning of the skin, fingernail changes, redness, or increased skin coloring and skin rash. Once in a while women experience dizziness, slurred speech, unsteadiness while walking, and uncontrolled eye movements. These end when treatment is over.

Precautions During Chemotherapy

Here are precautions to take while you are on chemotherapy:

- Unless you are wearing a mask, avoid indoor crowds when your white-blood-cell count is low.
- Avoid sick people.
- Eat only cooked fruits and vegetables when your white-blood-cell count is very low. (Absolute granulocyte count less than 1,000).
- If you run a temperature of 101 degrees or higher, you need to get a white-blood-cell count, and if it is low, you need to enter the hospital *immediately* for intravenous antibiotics.

While you are going through chemotherapy, medical personnel will carefully monitor your progress. You'll have frequent blood tests to watch for effects of the drug on your bone marrow.

Some people simply do not tolerate chemotherapy well, and it takes some trial and error to find the right treatment program for them, along with antinausea drugs to keep side effects at a minimum. With some chemotherapy drugs, nausea can be decreased or eliminated by giving the drugs as a prolonged continuous infusion (IV) rather than by rapid injection.

Nutritional Needs During Chemotherapy

You're probably going to get tired of people talking to you about nutrition while you are going through chemotherapy and recovering from cancer. But remember that you need to focus all of your body's weapons to fight this disease.

For your body to be its most effective, it must be strong. One component of strength is rest and another is nutrition. Research proves that well-nourished cancer patients withstand treatment better than malnourished patients.

The key is to follow a nutritious diet. That means getting a balance of food containing vitamins, minerals, proteins, and carbohydrates. To do so, select foods from the basic four groups:

- *Milk and milk products:* Milk, ice cream, cottage cheese, and cheese supply protein, calcium, and vitamins.
- *Poultry, fish, and meat:* Red meat may taste terrible to you right now, but you can also get protein from fish, chicken, and eggs. Vegetarians will want to increase their intake of beans and nuts. These foods also supply vitamins and minerals.
- *Fruits and vegetables:* These are an important source of vitamins and minerals and you may want to do some study about them and how they interact with the body. Green, leafy vegetables are especially important sources of needed nutrients.
- *Cereals and whole grains:* In addition to being an excellent source of nutrients, products made of corn, wheat, rice, and oats give you the roughage

that will help your digestive system function as normally as possible.

Good Nutrition Will Help You Get Well

As you learn more about nutrition, you'll view food as one of your weapons against cancer. Protein is especially important because it helps your body repair tissue and replace lost or injured cells. You also need to take in an appropriate number of calories.

If you are underweight, you may need to experiment with some various ways to get yourself to eat enough. Taking frequent walks, including a long one before each meal, might increase your appetite. Eating frequent small meals is another strategy that works for some people.

It Takes Work to Eat Right

This is a good time to explore bookstores to search out cookbooks with nutritious recipes and to spend a lot of time trying various recipes. If you find you have no interest at all in food and cannot face trying to cook, you may want to turn over this task to someone in your family or to a good friend.

You may find that sometimes you feel up to cooking and sometimes you don't. When you do, cook ahead, making quantities of food to eat on those days when you don't have the energy or interest to make food.

When you eat, eat slowly and chew your food carefully. That will help your stomach with digestion. Avoid fatty and fried foods. They're harder to digest and the smell of these foods cooking may nauseate you. Sometimes it helps to eat foods at room temperature instead of hot or chilled foods.

When in Doubt, Consult Your Doctor

You might be used to a glass of wine, a cocktail, or a beer before or with meals; during chemotherapy you may or may not have to give this up. Alcohol can interact with some medications, producing undesirable side effects or inhibiting the effectiveness of the chemotherapy. You'll need to discuss this with medical personnel who know which drugs you're taking and how alcohol reacts with them.

Finally, do not experiment with strange diets or megavitamin regimens during chemotherapy, no matter how strongly their anticancer properties may be touted. You need good, balanced nutrition, combined with plenty of rest and careful medical monitoring during this stressful time. Some vitamins in high doses may increase the side effects of your drugs or interfere with their cancer-killing activity. Do not take more than one all-purpose vitamin per day. Ask your doctor for guidance.

Warning Signs of Infection

Any changes in your health should be reported to your doctor. Signs of trouble include diarrhea, pain during urination, fever, chills, sweating, severe coughing, or a sore throat.

As we already noted, go to the doctor's office or hospital and get a blood test if you run a fever of 101 degrees or more. If your white-blood-cell count is low, you will need to begin antibiotics. And don't take aspirin without permission from your doctor.

Find Ways to Control Your Stress

No one else can really advise you on how to get control of your life at a time like this.

You may need help. A trusted friend, your spouse or lover, a relative, a volunteer from the American Cancer Society, members of an "I Can Cope" support group, or a professional counselor are all people who can help you and will probably gladly do so. But they must hear from you just what your needs are. No one can read your mind. Remember, most people *want* to help, and will be happy to do anything they can for you, whether it's cooking meals or helping out around the house, or taking long walks with you and talking about your concerns. Give them a chance!

Questions to Ask Your Doctor

- Am I a candidate for chemotherapy?
- What are the benefits and risks of the type of chemotherapy you are recommending?
- When will my chemotherapy begin and how long will it last?
- Where will I receive my treatments?
- How will I receive my treatments?
- What are the possible side effects during treatment?
- Do you know of any long-term effects?
- Are there any danger signs I should report to you?
- Will I be able to keep up with my regular activi-

ties, job, taking care of my children, etc., during chemotherapy?

- Are there any restrictions I should observe regarding food or activities?
- Do you know of any breast cancer volunteers or specially trained counselors to whom I can speak if I feel the need?

10 Hormone Therapy

This chapter, like the last, is quite technical, but we have tried to share the information women with breast cancer want.

When the biopsy was performed on the mass or lump first discovered in one of your breasts, the laboratory analysis on it included estrogen and progesterone receptor tests (or hormone receptor assays).

The pathologist overseeing the testing wanted to find out if your tumor contained *receptors* that allow estrogen to stimulate the cancer growth.

* * *

Hormone Receptors

About 60 percent of all women with breast cancer have tumors that contain greater than normal levels of estrogen and/or progesterone receptors. The more receptors a tumor contains, the more likely that growth is dependent on estrogen, and the more likely that the tumor growth can be arrested by being denied access to normal levels of estrogen.

The Positive and Negative Factor

Tumors that have a high concentration of estrogen receptors in their cells are referred to as estrogen receptor positive (ER+), and tumors that have very few or an undetectable number of estrogen receptors are referred to as estrogen receptive negative (ER−).

In the same way, tumors with high concentrations of progesterone receptors are referred to as progesterone receptor positive (PR+), and those with few receptors are referred to as progesterone receptor negative (PR−). Some women are both ER+ and PR+. The presence of both receptors usually means the hormone response mechanism is intact. Therefore, women who are both ER+ and PR+ have a better chance of responding to hormone treatment than women who are only ER+.

When breast cancer has spread beyond the breasts and into the underarm nodes or into the rest of the body, the cancerous cells usually have the same characteristics they had when present in the breast. They are still ER+ or ER−, and PR+ or PR−.

Hormone Therapy

With reliable hormone receptor tests to reveal this information, and with what researchers continue to learn about the interaction of hormones and hormone-dependent cells, they have developed an approach to breast cancer treatment called hormone therapy. Statistically, a tumor that is both ER+ and PR+ has an 80 percent chance of responding to hormone therapy.

Hormonal therapies actually prevent the cells from receiving or processing the normal hormones that stimulate their growth. This will cause the cancer cells to cease growing, and most will eventually die. Thus, "hormonal therapies" are actually anti-estrogen or antihormone treatments. There are many different types, but the commonly used adjuvant treatments are tamoxifen if the woman is peri-menopausal (close to menopause) or postmenopausal, and removing the ovaries if a woman is premenopausal.

Tamoxifen, the most commonly used adjuvant antihormonal therapy, works by competing with the body's estrogen for receptors on the surface of the cell. Once on the receptor, tamoxifen passes into the nucleus that gives instructions to the rest of the cell on how to operate. Part of the signal it gives is faulty, and as a result the cancer cell cannot easily divide and eventually dies.

To work, tamoxifen must be present in one hundred to one thousand times greater amounts than the estrogen in the body. Thus, tamoxifen does not always work well in younger premenopausal women, because with commonly used doses it often cannot compete with the levels of estrogen they produce. Tamoxifen signals the pituitary that more estrogen is needed, which causes the pituitary to signal the ovary to increase estrogen output. In the peri-menopausal and postmenopausal woman, this is not a problem because the ovaries are not able to increase estrogen output much in response to the pituitary signal.

For the young postmenopausal woman needing antihormone therapy, the most rational treatment in the past has been to remove the ovaries (oophorectomy). A new treatment, Zoladex, has been developed that blocks the pituitary signal to the ovaries and allows a woman to avoid surgery. Clinical trials with Zoladex and tamoxifen are now in progress.

Antihormone drugs may work only as long as they are given. Consequently, most women are now being advised to take them for five years or longer.

Drawbacks to Antihormone Treatment

The major drawback to antihormonal therapy is that the killing of cells may not be as complete as it is with chemotherapy because there are usually some cells within a tumor that have few or no hormone receptors. Antihormone treatments won't work well on these. Also, some cancer cells will not die when given antihormone treatments, but will instead go into a prolonged inactive state.

Tamoxifen, the most frequently used adjuvant antihormone treatment, can cause side effects that include weight gain, fluid retention, hot flashes, vaginal discharge, headaches, and depression, and an increased tendency to form gallstones. In addition, tamoxifen, like estrogen, causes a slightly increased risk of endometrial cancer in women who have not had a hysterectomy.

Tamoxifen also causes an increased risk of blood clots in leg veins.

Advantages of Antihormone Drugs

Antihormone drugs have far fewer side effects than chemotherapy. There is no hair loss or danger of infection, and the incidence of nausea and vomiting is markedly lower.

Tamoxifen may offer some benefits for postmenopausal women, including lowering cholesterol and protection against osteoporosis (bone loss). It may also help suppress new tumor growth in the opposite breast.

Candidates for Hormone Treatments

Hormone treatments usually only work well in women who have large amounts of estrogen and progesterone receptors in their tumors, and whose tumors are growing slowly (low S-phase). This is particularly true in older, postmenopausal women.

Women whose tumors are ER– or who have low-to-intermediate amounts of estrogen and progesterone receptors, or whose tumors are poorly differentiated or are growing quickly (high S-phase), will probably not do well with hormone treatment alone.

These women should receive chemotherapy as the mainstay of their treatment. If the tumor is ER+, however, antihormone therapy can be added once the chemotherapy is completed.

Standard Hormonal Treatments

The standard treatment for postmenopausal women who are strongly ER+ or PR+ is tamoxifen alone, either taken indefinitely or for a minimum of five years.

There is no standard hormone therapy for premenopausal women who are strongly ER+ or PR+. Standard treatment in the United States for these women is chemotherapy.

Combination Hormonal and Chemotherapy: A Look to the Future

Preliminary studies have indicated that some types of chemotherapy agents may be useful adjuncts to hormonal therapy in some postmenopausal ER+ patients. This may be particularly true in women with fast-growing or poorly differentiated tumors.

Likewise, adjuvant hormonal treatment may be beneficial to some ER+ premenopausal women taking chemotherapy.

Why not just give both at the same time to everybody?

It's not that simple. If the tumor was initially growing rapidly, hormone therapy can slow down the growth rate of the tumor and make the cells harder to kill with drugs. In postmenopausal patients with a very slow-growing ER+ tumor, adding chemotherapy to the tamoxifen may only add side effects and expense. In addition, there is a much higher risk of developing blood clots in the large veins of the legs and pelvis when both treatments are given together than when either is given alone.

We are also beginning to discover that aside from growth rate, tamoxifen and other antihormones may favorably influence the killing action of some chemotherapy drugs (e.g., Adriamycin) and cause problems with others.

Needless to say, combination adjuvant hormonal treatments and chemotherapy is still a subject of considerable controversy.

In general, caution should be exercised in the simultaneous administration of tamoxifen and many types of chemotherapy because tamoxifen can interfere with their tumor-killing effects.

However, for women who are strongly ER+, whose tumors are rapidly growing, and who are not study candidates, considerations should be given to indefinite hormonal treatment following chemotherapy. For post- or peri-menopausal women (naturally, surgically, or chemotherapy-induced), the hormonal treatment of choice would be tamoxifen.

For young premenopausal women having regular periods after chemotherapy, the hormonal treatment of choice would be oophorectomy or Zoladex plus tamoxifen.

Hormonal Replacement

Research is currently under way to discover safe ways to avoid hot flashes, vaginal dryness, and skin changes that result from estrogen loss. Estrogen can stimulate growth of any estrogen receptor positive cancer cells remaining in your body. Since most estrogen receptor negative tumors have some estrogen receptor

positive cells, even women with estrogen receptor negative tumors should avoid oral, vaginal, or any other type
of estrogen replacement if the breast cancer has a sub-
stantial chance of recurrence and/or breast tissue remains.

We don't know exactly how long women should
avoid estrogen replacement, but since breast cancer can
recur even ten years or more after surgery, one needs to
avoid estrogen indefinitely if there is remaining breast
tissue or a significant chance of tumor recurrence elsewhere in the body.

What Can I Safely Do About Hot Flashes?

If you are experiencing hot flashes, there are several
things you can do to decrease the severity. These include
wearing loose-fitting cotton or other natural-fiber clothing and experimenting with several different types of
medicine, including Clonidine (patch or pill), Bellergal,
and Thorazine. An antidepressant such as Elavil may
help you sleep better at night and avoid some of the
mood swings that accompany the hormonal changes associated with hot flashes.

Like chemotherapy and so many other medical facts
related to breast cancer and its treatment, hormone
therapy is difficult to understand. Many of the terms are
technical and complicated sounding. But you need to be
part of your own treatment team and you need to understand not only what is happening to you, but how you
are being treated.

Don't shy away from asking medical personnel to
explain things in language you can understand. Seek to
know exactly what is going on!

Hormone therapy is a field of constant discovery

and change. You may not be able to find all the information you need in this chapter. If that happens, be sure to ask your doctors for clear answers.

Questions to Ask Your Doctor

- Am I a candidate for hormone therapy?
- If so, what are the risks of the therapy you recommend?
- What are the potential side effects?
- If there are side effects, are there ways they can be treated or minimized?
- How long will I be on this program?
- Will it be combined with any other course of treatment? If so, why?

<u>11</u> Physical Therapy

Less than a decade ago, when the radical and modified radical mastectomy were the usual surgical options for breast cancer, physical recovery was a major ordeal.

Skin tightening, scarring, and arm swelling following removal of some of the chest muscles, skin, axillary lymph nodes and tissue frequently limited recovering full use of the arm and shoulder.

Today, with less drastic forms of surgery, physical recovery usually goes much more smoothly.

Still, any kind of surgery that affects the chest wall and the underarm can cause complications, as can radiation therapy. For these reasons, you may want to consider some specialized physical therapy.

Assessment Before Surgery Will Help

Once you learn that you will have a mastectomy or lumpectomy, it can be very helpful to visit an occupational therapist (O.T.) or physical therapist (P.T.) for baseline testing. The therapist will perform a series of tests on you, determining the range of motion for your arm and shoulder so you will know what to strive for after surgery. By measuring the circumference of your arm, the therapist will know through subsequent measurements after surgery if you are developing lymphedema (there is a discussion of lymphedema later in this chapter).

The therapist will also want to know if you have any particular problems with your neck, arm, or shoulder, such as any past injuries that still trouble you. Such information will be helpful in developing a good useful exercise program for you.

If you don't have the opportunity to visit with a therapist before surgery, test the range of motion of your arm and shoulder on yourself so you can strive to attain it again after surgery. If you have had a neck, shoulder, or arm injury sometime in the past, be sure to mention this to your doctor when you discuss post-op exercise.

Physical Therapy After Surgery

As soon as the tissue around your incision is healed, your doctor will give you clearance to begin some simple exercises. You'll want to do these because they will help you regain your strength and prevent weakness from developing in your affected arm.

It's a natural reaction after surgery to "favor" the affected area, putting as little stress and strain on it as possible. But after breast cancer surgery, it's important to begin using your arm just as much as you can. If you refuse to use the arm, the shoulder joint will become severely limited in its range of motion. This is often referred to as a "frozen" shoulder. The older you are, the more danger there is of developing a frozen shoulder.

You'll want to continue with special exercises for at least a year following surgery. If you have an implanted catheter, it's important that you take special precautions not to disturb it.

If you visited an O.T. or P.T. before your surgery for baseline testing, return as soon after surgery as possible for further assessment and to work out an exercise program geared just to you and your needs. If that's not possible, you can do exercises on your own that will help you regain your strength and also reduce pain and stiffness in your neck and back, should these trouble you.

Special Exercises Help Greatly

The National Cancer Institute recommends the following exercises, beginning them shortly after surgery:

- Lying in bed, position the affected arm at your side. Raise it straight up and back, trying to touch the headboard.
- Loosen your chest, shoulders, and upper back muscles by raising your shoulders and then rotating them forward, down, and back in a circular motion.
- Push your elbows into the mattress as you lie in bed and clasp your hands behind your head.

- Bend your elbow and arm at a ninety-degree angle to your body. Rotate your shoulder forward and backward.
- Raise your arm, then clench and unclench your fist.
- Breathe deeply.
- Rotate your chin to the left and the right. Cock your head sideways.

Special Programs Are Also Helpful

If you are visited by a Reach to Recovery volunteer while you are in the hospital, she may bring you a set of exercises and also show you how to do them.

If you live near a YWCA, you may want to find out if they have an ENCORE program. This is an exercise and discussion program for women who have had breast cancer. Often it's organized around swimming, walking, and light aerobics. You'll probably find that the combination of exercise and conversation is especially therapeutic.

If no such program exists, you might want to seek out one or two swimming or walking partners who have been through your experience and form your own little support group.

While you don't want to overdo your exercise, you want to do enough. You should not engage in any stretching exercise that causes severe pain in the chest or arm or marked shortness of breath, or that raises the pulse over the maximum exercise heart rate recommended for your age.

*   *   *

Lymphedema

Physicians don't see nearly as much of this condition as they did when radical and modified mastectomies were the norm, but it can still occur. Lymphedema is a chronic swelling of the hand and arm. Lymph vessels resemble veins. They carry fluid and white blood cells from the peripheral tissues of the hand and arm. The lymph channels periodically empty into nodes and eventually empty into the bloodstream in the chest by way of the thoracic duct.

Following axillary lymph node dissection, with or without radiation, these lymph channels can become scarred and obliterated, and then fluid cannot be carried away as efficiently from the tissues. As a consequence, the arm and shoulder area can become quite swollen and sore.

Arm infections occur more frequently in women with lymphedema. If the arm becomes acutely red and generally more swollen, or if red streaks are seen traveling up the arm, be sure to report them to your doctor. Older women are more at risk for this condition because their skin and tissue have lost some of their elasticity.

If you do experience some swelling, you'll want to follow some simple rules until it's under control:

- Avoid wearing anything that puts pressure on the arm, wrist, or shoulder.
- Do not carry heavy objects or handbags with the affected hand and arm.
- Be very careful not to cut yourself near the affected area. A nick with a razor, a thorn prick with a rose, or any other kind of cut can cause a seri-

169

ous infection. Avoid having blood drawn from that arm.

The Pneumatic Pump

In order to clear up lymphedema, your doctor may prescribe diuretics. You may also be a candidate for a procedure called pneumomassage. If so, you will go to the rehabilitation department in a hospital or a special rehabilitation center where a long sleeve that resembles the cuff used in taking your blood pressure will be wrapped around your arm. It is hooked up to the pneumatic pump machine. Via pressure, the massage action of the wrap forces the excess fluid in your arm back into the bloodstream.

When as much fluid as possible has been pumped out, you will be fitted for a Jobst stocking. This is a specially designed garment that fits over the affected arm and shoulder and through gentle pressure helps return lymph fluid to the major channels in the chest. It's like the special stockings worn by people who have severe varicose veins in their legs.

You'll continue with the pneumatic pump treatments for the next several days until the Jobst stocking arrives. The therapist will help you fit it and you will be instructed to put it on before getting up in the morning and to wear it until bedtime. You'll need to continue wearing the stocking until the lymphedema clears up, which could take weeks, months, or even longer.

Physical Therapy Can Help You Recover Faster

If you can do so, try to see an occupational or physical therapist after your surgery to discuss your recovery and any need you have for special assistance. A therapist will have many good suggestions for you on how to prevent injury to your affected arm and how to strengthen it.

Full recovery after any type of breast cancer surgery is contingent upon full physical recovery. Initially, special exercises may be painful, but they won't hurt you, and they will help you physically recover.

It's important that you do them faithfully. You may have to force yourself to stay with them—especially if you don't feel well and if you are having any problems with depression. But in the long run you will feel better both mentally and physically if you fully recover the strength and dexterity in your arm and shoulder that you had prior to surgery.

Questions to Ask Your Doctor

- Do you recommend that I see an occupational therapist or physical therapist before and/or after my surgery?
- What kind of exercise program do you suggest I follow?
- Who will teach me the exercises?
- What are signs of lymphedema that I should be aware of?
- How do you treat lymphedema?

171

12 Second Opinions, Miracle Cures

As you already know, much needs to be learned about cancer. In spite of ongoing research that increases our knowledge every day, much about cancer and its causes, treatments, and cures is still speculative.

It's very important that you, as a cancer patient, become actively involved in your own treatment. Not only should you understand exactly what's happening to you and have a say in treatment choices, you should also seek out sound medical advice. This may involve getting second opinions along the way. It also means opting for conventional medical treatment and undergoing carefully formulated procedures rather than resorting to promises of too-good-to-be-true cures you may hear about.

Seeking a Second Opinion

Many patients don't want a second opinion. They feel comfortable with their physicians and do not wish to take an active part in treatment selection. They may become frustrated, angry, tearful, or confused if presented with a variety of choices or detailed explanations of choices made for them.

Others go to the opposite extreme. They constantly challenge their physicians, demanding an explanation for each and every thing related to their care. They are often hostile toward everyone in the medical community and assume an attitude of "me against them." Rather than viewing medical personnel as friends, they view them as individuals not necessarily likely to have their best interests at heart, and hence they have difficulty trusting them. This attitude may be part of their overall personality or may be the result of previous experience with another physician.

As discussed in Chapter Two, the best place to be is between these two extremes. Be informed and involved in what's happening to you and in making decisions about your care. When you don't understand something or you're unsure of something, ask questions. Be pleasant to medical personnel and don't be afraid to express your feelings when you are troubled. Do not continue to be treated by a physician you do not feel comfortable with. You will make both of your lives miserable.

If you follow these guidelines, you will be the type of patient who receives the best care. You will be aware, informed, and reasonable.

Doctors Also Get Second Opinions

Much controversy exists in the cancer treatment field, and sometimes a different physician might suggest something the first one didn't know about or hadn't thought about. When there are several possible methods of treatment, get a second opinion if you are not quite comfortable with the suggested course of action.

There are two times especially when, as a breast cancer patient, you may want to seek a second opinion. The first time might be when you're deciding what type of surgical procedure is best for you. The second time is when deciding whether you need chemotherapy or hormone therapy following surgery, and what type might be best.

Good Doctors Aren't Offended

Don't worry that your doctor will be offended when you request referral to another doctor for a second opinion. Doctors are used to this, and most will willingly make such referrals. After all, they often render second opinions for other physicians.

If your attitude is friendly and professional and you assume it's a matter of course that you will seek a second opinion, your doctor should have no trouble with it. If he or she seems offended, you may want to select a different doctor. Your health is the most important thing here, and a second opinion may not only net you the best care, but will also set your mind at ease.

You may be pleasantly surprised to learn that your insurance company will pay for a second opinion. In fact, many insurance companies insist on second opinions before any surgical procedure.

If your doctor refuses to give you any names for referral, find another physician on your own by consulting medical directories, the American Cancer Society, medical centers, cancer hotlines, or calling other doctors' practices.

What If the Opinions Conflict?

When you get a second opinion and it's different from the first, then consider getting a third opinion. That doctor will likely agree with one of the other two, and you can go with the majority opinion. Do not be concerned if the suggested treatment differences are minor. There is still much disagreement among breast cancer specialists regarding many points of breast cancer treatment.

Important issues for invasive breast cancer are:

(1) Lumpectomy versus mastectomy.
(2) Whether or not to sample tissue from the opposite breast.
(3) Whether or not adjuvant (prophylactic) treatment of some kind is indicated.
(4) If adjuvant treatment is indicated, whether hormone therapy or chemotherapy or both is most appropriate.

The optimal type of chemotherapy to be administered and the exact length of time to administer it will depend on the age and physical condition of the patient, tumor characteristics, social considerations, physician preferences, where the physician trained, and whether or not you choose to be treated as part of a protocol or study.

Drug treatment is a field of active study, and your medical team will know the latest and best drugs and combinations that are suitable for you. Currently, chemotherapy lasts six to twelve months. The longer and more aggressive treatments may be indicated for women with large numbers of involved lymph nodes.

If you need hormone treatment, tamoxifen is the current drug of choice for postmenopausal women. It should be taken for a minimum of five to ten years, and possibly for life.

Important issues for noninvasive breast cancer or carcinoma in situ are:

(1) Lumpectomy without radiation, versus lumpectomy with radiation, versus mastectomy.
(2) Sampling tissue and/or treatment of the opposite breast.

If the area of carcinoma in situ is small and there is no immediate family history of breast cancer, most cancer specialists feel that lumpectomy with radiation to the tumor bed only is all that is required.

If the in situ carcinoma is large, then removal of the entire tumor, followed by whole-breast radiation or mastectomy with or without immediate reconstruction would currently be the procedures of choice. If multiple sites of in situ carcinoma are present throughout the breast, mastectomy would be best.

Lobular carcinoma in situ carries the same risk of developing invasive breast cancer in the opposite breast as the one in which the cancer was detected. This is not true for ductal carcinoma in situ, which often only occurs in one breast. The opposite breast should always be

177

sampled in patients with lobular carcinoma in situ. If mastectomy is chosen as a means of control, then it should be bilateral with bilateral immediate reconstruction if possible, and if the woman desires it.

As long as the carcinoma is noninvasive, it will not spread to the rest of the body. Only 50 percent of in situ carcinomas are associated with the later development of invasive cancer following biopsy.

Doctors Seek Second Opinions, Too

As discussed earlier in this book, many doctors seek second opinions before recommending a treatment plan for their breast cancer patients. Knowing how important their decisions are to their patients' health, they, too, want to be assured that they've made the absolutely best choice.

The American Medical Association's principles of medical ethics instruct physicians to consult with other physicians upon request in doubtful or difficult cases. In some hospitals, consultation of this sort is actually mandatory. The hospital may have established what they refer to as a tumor board. All new cases are brought up for review and the treatment plan is discussed by a group of professionals working together.

Remember, seeking a second opinion shows that you care enough about your own health to confirm what you are told.

What About Those Miracle Cures?

P. T. Barnum told us there's a sucker born every minute, and he knew what he was talking about.

Whether it's someone trying to sell you the Brooklyn Bridge, a gold mine in South America, or a "miracle" cure for cancer, the woods are full of frauds.

When it comes to cancer, people are desperate for cures. Standard treatments can be extreme, painful, and can't promise cure. It's no wonder so many people look for whatever hope they can find—and end up not only without a miracle cure, but also much poorer in the process. (As a society, we spend an estimated *two to three billion dollars* on unproven cancer treatments each year!)

Perhaps the greatest danger is that people will try fraudulent cures in place of standard treatment and lose vital time in their war against cancer.

Don't Trust Claims Because They're in the News

As stressful as breast cancer is, you don't need the added indignity of knowing you've lost your money to a charlatan who's convinced you that a special diet, special charm, special program, special water, special medicine, or whatever, will cure you. Look for the weaknesses in any claim, *even if you read about it in a newspaper article.*

Why can't you trust what you read in the newspaper? Because often newspapers (and magazines and television) circulate a story that has no scientific basis. Read the article or listen to the news spot carefully. If the results are from a scientific journal and are based on controlled studies, then they are probably accurate. But if the report is from a doctor or lay group that has made some sort of claim without being published in a reputable medical journal, they probably don't have the scientific data to back their claim. Remember—anyone can claim to be an expert. Anyone can send out a press release, and the media may report it without doing any checking.

If a service or product can actually cure cancer, you can be certain that the scientific community will quickly zero in on it. Most scientists would like nothing better than to see cancer eliminated in our lifetimes, and if any claim merits their attention, it will get it.

As with any "miracle" cure, look at claims to cure breast cancer with a wary eye. If it promises to be simple, painless, and effective, and if it sounds too good to be true, you can be certain that it is.

Questions to Ask About Second Opinions

- Has my case already been presented at a tumor board or conference?
- If not, can you recommend another specialist I can see to get a second opinion?

Questions to Ask Regarding "Miracle" Cures

- Is this claim based on controlled studies?
- Why hasn't this treatment been reported in scientific or medical journals?
- Does this treatment have endorsement from qualified medical personnel?
- What kind of guarantee does this treatment have? Will actual people vouch for it—or does it adver-

tise itself with terms like, "millions of people have been cured"?

- How much does this treatment cost?
- Can I actually speak to someone who has been cured of breast cancer as a result of this service or product?
- Does this claim sound too good to be true?

13 Recovering Physically from Cancer

Recovering your physical health is yet another mountain to climb when you have breast cancer. As tough as the experiences of needle aspiration, biopsy, surgery, chemotherapy, radiation, and hormone therapy can be, coping with your day-to-day health needs is also a challenge.

Ideally, you will invest your time and resources in leading as stress-free and healthy a life as possible. You'll make yourself your number-one priority and concentrate on taking care of yourself. Your friends and family will handle all of life's nitty-gritty for you, leaving you free to attend to yourself and your needs.

In reality, it probably won't work that way. If you have a family, and especially if you have young children, you may face a barrage of "must do's" almost from the moment you get home from the hospital. If, on top of everything else, you have a demanding job, you may have very little time to think about taking care of yourself.

The Importance of Taking Care of Yourself

But you must. Attending to the needs of your physical self is critical to your recovery. (We'll cover taking care of your emotional self in the next section of this book.) Your body has gone through a very traumatic experience. Whether you had a lumpectomy or a mastectomy, recovering from surgery requires that every component of your body and mind join forces to make you healthy again.

If you are undergoing radiation and/or chemotherapy, your body has even more work to do. Not only must you recover physically from the surgery, but because treatment temporarily depletes your white cells, you are susceptible to infection and must take precautions. On top of it all, you may feel fatigued. Perhaps you're also experiencing diarrhea, constipation, nausea, and vomiting. Treatment can also change your looks, causing dry or irritated skin and scalp. If you are receiving chemotherapy, having your hair fall out can be the final blow.

Put Your Own Needs First

With all these physical complications, eating right, getting enough sleep and exercise, and doing everything you can to eliminate stress are vitally important. For a while, at least, you must put your own needs first. If you can't make your family and employer understand the importance of this, ask your doctor to assist you in getting the word to them. Chances are he or she has done this before with other families and employers and, knowing that this is critical, will readily do it for you.

The Importance of Good Nutrition While Recovering from Cancer

With all the information that is available to us about health and nutrition, most of us know that our bodies depend upon food for energy and strength.

America is a society of junk-food addicts, and many people don't have the habit of eating foods that are nutritious and good for them. Instead, they are addicted to the salt, fat, and sugar that flavor greasy burgers and fries. Those aren't the ingredients that are going to help you get well. Nutritious foods are the ones your mother and grandmother told you to eat—fresh fruits, vegetables, dairy products, lean meat and fish, and whole-grain breads. You also need to drink lots of water.

Educate Yourself About Nutrition

Your period of recovery from cancer may have to be a time of retraining yourself to eat foods that are good for you and will assist you in regaining your health. As we suggested earlier, you may want to spend some time in a good bookstore or at the library, educating yourself about nutrition and what foods constitute a healthy diet.

For example, while dairy foods are generally good for you, too much butter or too many eggs are not. While meat and fish are good for you, eating them fried or coated with batter and then baked or fried is not. Whole-grain bread is good for you—but not if you top it with globs of butter or sugary jelly.

If you're going through radiation, you may need more than the usual number of calories because your body is burning up energy at an increased rate in order to replace and repair the white cells that have been damaged. But you still need to exercise caution as to how you take them into your body.

If you are receiving chemotherapy or hormone therapy, you may not need any more calories, and may possibly need fewer calories than you normally do.

Many women are overweight when they develop breast cancer and have the mistaken idea that chemotherapy is synonymous with weight loss. It's not. In fact, probably due to the suppressive effects of chemotherapy on ovarian function, as well as decreased physical activity, many women gain ten to twenty pounds. Many also gain weight on tamoxifen for the same reasons, especially if they were peri-menopausal when the tamoxifen was started.

Getting the Most Nutritional Value from Daily Calories

Make certain that what you're eating is good for you. Healthy sources of calories are peanut butter, honey, sour cream, yogurt, milk, ice cream, and raisins, dates, and nuts. If swallowing is a problem for you, in the special foods section of your grocery store or at health-food stores you'll find high-calorie liquid protein supplements that offer the advantage of liquid smoothness.

You Need All Types of Foods

Protein is a nutrient you'll want to pay special attention to. It helps repair body tissue and will assist your skin, hair, muscles, and tissue in their return to their normal state. Meat, fish, poultry, eggs, and cheese are good protein sources. Make sure the meat is lean and that you discard the skin of the chicken in order to eliminate unhealthy fat from these otherwise protein-rich foods. Meat, you'll recall, is one of the four basic food groups, and our body benefits from at least one daily serving.

Fresh fruits and vegetables, the second major food group, will supply you with vitamins and minerals and also some protein. This might be a good time to invest in a juice extractor so you can experiment in drinking the juices of these healthy foods. Again, this can be helpful if swallowing is difficult for you.

Milk products—milk, yogurt, cheese, eggs, cottage cheese, sour cream, and ice cream—are important sources of protein and calcium. They are the third major food group.

The fourth basic food group is grains. This group includes rice, pasta, cereal, and bread. Once again, go for as pure a product as possible. Grains supply vitamins, minerals, some protein, and fiber. Fiber assists the digestive tract by helping to move food through the intestines and out of the body.

For grain products to be nutritionally superior, select those made with unrefined flour and whole grains. Cakes, rolls, and white breads made with highly processed and refined flours have lost much of their nutritional benefits. Cooked cereals like oatmeal are also very good sources of grain fiber.

Finally, drink lots of water. It helps the body maintain its proper fluid balance. If you don't get enough water, you may feel tired and may get headaches.

Get Plenty of Sleep

If you have a job outside the home, and if you also have young children, getting enough sleep may be another major challenge for you. Your period of recovery from cancer is a time when you not only need a full night of sleep—seven to eight hours—but may well need a couple of additional hours per night as well. Even with that, fatigue may be an ongoing problem, especially if you're receiving radiation and/or chemotherapy.

Your body will tell you how much sleep it needs, and the wisest thing you could do is to listen to it and give it this amount. Make no apology for this. Your system is working overtime, and it's very important work that it's doing. You'll have to plan other components of life around this for at least a few months.

Exercise Will Help You Feel Good

As we stated earlier, if you receive chemotherapy or hormone therapy, you may probably gain ten to twenty pounds. Exercise will help prevent this weight gain—or help take it off once it's on. Exercise also releases chemicals called endorphins that help you feel better about yourself. Before you begin a strenuous fitness program, talk it over with your doctor. No one, however, will object to low-impact aerobics.

A daily walk is actually one of the best things you can do for yourself. In the beginning you may not feel like doing anything more than walking a half block. Gradually you'll not only find you want to go farther, but you'll probably look forward to the outing. Fresh air will make you feel good, and it's good for you. It will help stimulate your appetite and help you sleep better. It will also help control stress, and it will help you get and keep your body fit.

Gentle stretching exercises will limber up your body each morning so that muscles won't feel tight and achy. As we discussed in Chapter Eleven, if you've had a mastectomy, you'll want to continue to exercise your chest and arm area until they are completely healed. You may even want to do some mild lifting exercises with hand weights.

Get on Top of Stress

Your body will heal faster if you can control stress. Medical experts are learning more all the time about the effect of stress on the body. It can be devastating, to the point of actually causing people to become ill.

Of course you feel stress right now. Your body has all these extra needs at a time when you don't feel well. You've taken time off work for surgery and treatment and may be running out of sick leave. Your family's needs continue apace, and they don't understand why you can't do the things you always did for them. The medical bills and insurance forms are piling up and need attention. You and your husband or lover may not be communicating very well. Your hair may be falling out. You've lost a breast—an integral part of your feminine self—and must come to terms with that. And on top of it all, you're wondering if there's a possibility that your cancer may return.

Talk about stress! How you control it is an individual matter. People will try to advise you, but you must find the solution that works best for you.

It may be a long walk first thing in the morning or in the middle of the day or in the evening—or all three. It may be attending a workout center or taking a yoga class.

It may be attending support groups for cancer patients, such as "I Can Cope," or spending time with friends and family members, just talking.

It may be prayer or meditation or writing in a journal. Or it may be seeing a counselor—a minister, social worker, psychologist, or psychiatrist—who can help you work through and express your feelings.

The worst thing you can do is push yourself immediately to be "back to normal." That will only lead to physical exhaustion. Listen to your body—and give it what it needs.

Follow-up Doctor Visits

Most women find their frequent checkups with their doctor to be especially stressful because they fear they'll hear more bad news. As hard as it may be to go, don't put it off. You need regular and thorough medical care to catch any arising problems as quickly as possible and to monitor your health-care program.

If you are receiving chemotherapy, you will probably be monitored by a medical oncologist. Otherwise, your checkups may be through your family doctor or surgeon. In the beginning, you'll be on a frequent schedule of office visits. Initially your doctor will check the breast area and your incision, and will discuss how you're feeling and the state of your overall health.

You'll have a physical exam and blood work done every few months. You may also have a chest X ray and a bone scan done once a year for the first few years after surgery, depending on the risk of recurrence. You should always have a mammogram of the remaining breast performed yearly.

Concern About Recurrence

We know that 60 percent of all recurrences of breast cancer occur within the first three years after treatment, so this is a critical time. While you have possibly heard that if you pass the five-year mark without recurrence, you are given a clean bill of health, this is not entirely accurate. Certainly you can be quite optimistic at that point, but you'll want to be vigilant for another ten to fifteen years.

Symptoms you should report to a physician are:

- Lumps, thickenings, or inflammation in either breast or in your scar.
- Loss of appetite, persistent dizziness, headaches, or blurred vision.
- Persistent pain somewhere in the body, especially the back or ribs.
- Coughing or hoarseness that won't go away.

If You Move Away from Your Physician

If you move away from your primary-care physician, reestablish yourself with a new doctor right away.

191

Because your new doctor may want to speak with your former doctor or doctors, share all your records and medical information.

At the time of your move, inform your doctor and the medical center where you had your surgery and any kind of treatment. Your present doctor may be able to recommend a new doctor to you.

Make sure that before you move you have a copy of a dictated treatment summary, operative reports, pathology reports, and special test reports on the tumor. Also get copies of your chemotherapy flow sheets or records and X-ray reports. You may also want a film copy of your last mammogram. You may have to pay for some of these items, but they are important and the cost will be worth it.

With this information in hand, you can be assured that your new physician will understand what has happened to you.

Monthly Breast Self-Exam

Your monthly breast self-exam is still very important. If you are menstruating, the best time for this is two or three days after your period ends. If you are not menstruating, then the important thing is that you pick a regular time for your self-exam so you don't forget to do it. As an example, some women make it a routine on the first of every month.

After radiation, breast tissue often feels different than it did before treatment, so you'll have to get used to what the new feeling is like in order to know if something feels different.

If you're not familiar with how to do a breast self-exam, your physician or a member of his or her medical staff will show you how.

If You Have a Sister or Daughter

In the event that you have a sister or daughter, they should be advised to be very meticulous about performing breast self-exam on themselves and in getting regular mammograms after age thirty along with regular checkups.

Because of the known genetic link in breast cancer, they are at increased risk. They should begin getting screening mammograms ten years before the age that your cancer was discovered, even if this means that they start before age thirty.

The more they know and the more careful they are, the better. In spite of all we *don't* know about breast cancer, one thing we know for certain is that the earlier it's caught, the better are your chances for full physical recovery.

While your body will never be quite the same again, particularly if you've had a mastectomy, you *can* regain your physical health. You may even find that you feel better than ever, knowing you have faced a tremendous challenge. But reaching this state depends on you and your commitment to being as healthy as you can be. You'll find the benefits to be worth far more than whatever effort you must invest.

Questions to Ask Your Doctor

- What nutrition and exercise guidelines do you recommend that I follow?

- If I don't feel like eating, what do you suggest?
- How often should I have follow-up checkups?
- Will your office call me, or should I schedule them myself?
- What tests will you perform?
- Is there anything about my particular situation that would affect how I do breast self-examination?

II Emotional Recovery

INTRODUCTION

As difficult as the physical recovery from breast cancer can be, for most women the emotional recovery is also a special challenge.

Given how many women contract breast cancer, you know that survivors are all around you and that each one has her own special story. Here are the personal battles against breast cancer of four women.

Elaine

Elaine found out on her twenty-fifth wedding anniversary that a routine mammogram showed something suspicious. When she learned she would have a mastectomy, she decided to have immediate breast reconstruction. Tissue expanders were put in place at the time of her mastectomy.

The surgery seemed easy compared with what followed. Because of fluid accumulation, the reconstructed breast area had to be aspirated several times in the ensuing weeks. This resulted in a bacterial infection in the reconstructed breast, and the expanders had to be removed. During the two weeks it took her to recover, she was unable to start her chemotherapy. This frightened her because she had lymph node involvement and had been told it was important to start as soon as possible.

When she did start, she got her heavy dark hair cut very short. Three weeks later almost all of it fell out.

"That was such a humiliating experience," she recalled. "It was almost worse than losing a breast. I'd always had great hair. I could hide a missing breast behind a T-shirt, but what do you do with a bald head?"

Elaine disliked wearing a wig, so what she chose to do was to work with what hair she had left and to pay a great deal of attention to how she dressed. She visited ethnic clothing stores and started to sew and was soon wearing dramatic, colorful outfits with matching wraps on her head.

"I learned how to stuff two shoulder pads under a turban to make it look as though it had hair underneath it. That actually made my very serious oncologist laugh, and I enjoyed that. Every week when I went for chemo, it was a fashion show. The nurses couldn't wait to see what I would be wearing. I even made turbans for some of them.

"I found it very depressing to sit in that waiting room surrounded by women wearing no makeup who had terrycloth hats on their bald heads. I just had to do something."

Because Elaine's two daughters were grown and she didn't work outside the home, she knew that she had to keep busy or she would isolate herself and feel sorry for herself. When she wasn't working on outfits, she kept busy in other ways. She baked muffins for her elderly neighbors and cookies for the medical staff.

She and her husband, Chuck, an advertising director, stayed socially active. "I was fortunate that I didn't have to have radiation and I felt fairly good while I was on chemo," she said. "Twelve months of chemo. I call it my cancer year. I haven't decided yet if I'll go through reconstruction. I don't like wearing a prosthesis, so maybe I will. I reserve that decision for the future."

Elaine credits a good husband, her faith in God, and

her sense of humor for helping her through her cancer year.

"How do people get through an experience like this without faith?" she wondered. "You've got to have something to hold you together. And you've got to stay busy."

Beverly

Beverly wanted to stay busy during her cancer treatment, but didn't feel well enough to work in her real-estate and insurance agency.

"I think the year I was on chemo I was functioning at about 40 percent," she said. "I felt sick all the time and I was always tired. But I forced myself to work as much as I could, and that helped. I didn't give myself time to dwell on my fears. I made myself go on, even though it was often a challenge."

Beverly, who's fifty-six, had a routine mammogram two weeks after a routine doctor's exam. She was shocked to learn she had a lump because she had never worried about breast cancer.

"My sister died of colon cancer, and I had a pre-cancerous condition of the uterus and cervix that I was being treated for, so breast cancer never occurred to me," she said. "When I found out I had it, I was fatalistic. I just figured that was the beginning of the end since my sister had died of cancer."

Beverly had a double mastectomy and a year of chemotherapy. There was no node involvement. She has since had reconstruction, a process she's not certain she would go through again, knowing what she now knows.

"I live in a small town and I had to make dozens of trips to the city for medical appointments," she said. "By the time it was all over, I just felt I'd been through too much surgery."

Wearing a wig after her hair fell out didn't present a problem for her. "I had a good one and wearing it made me feel a little less freaky. My hair came back grayer than before, but otherwise the same. I viewed losing my hair as a sign that the chemo was working. It had to be, as sick as it made me.

"Whenever I felt sorry for myself, I'd think of the young woman I knew who was going through the same thing as me. She was only thirty-two and hadn't had children yet. And her cancer was more advanced than mine."

Betsy

Betsy is a college professor who teaches the sociology of medicine to medical students at a large medical center. Her specialty is terminal illness.

"There's a coping phenomenon among very ill people called 'downward comparison,'" she said. "You compare yourself to others. Someone with Lou Gehrig's disease looks at someone with multiple sclerosis and says, 'Thank God I'm not that helpless. The person with multiple sclerosis looks at the Lou Gehrig patient and says, 'At least I have twenty years to live.' They both look at cancer patients and say, 'At least I don't have that pain.' As a cancer patient, what I said was, 'At least I've got a whole arsenal of weapons to fight this disease. Because it's amazing what can be done to help cancer patients today."

Betsy, forty-seven, found the rapidly growing lump in her breast just one month after a physical exam had declared her fine. The biopsy showed cancer and the surgeon she consulted recommended a lumpectomy followed by both internal and external radiation.

During surgery, lymph node involvement was discovered, so adjuvant chemotherapy was recommended. She started radiation.

At the time Betsy was having a Hickman catheter put on the other side of her chest to deliver the chemotherapy, her oncologist recommended doing a "mirror image" biopsy of the opposite breast. (Mirror image biopsies involve removing a piece of tissue from the area of the "healthy" breast that corresponds to the place where cancer was found in the diseased breast. Mirror image biopsies are recommended when conditions suggest a high probability of two primary breast cancers.) The mirror image biopsy revealed a secondary cancer. Because of this new development, Betsy underwent a bilateral mastectomy, followed by nine months of chemotherapy.

"I've always been real energetic, but while I was on chemo I had low-grade nausea and hardly any energy," she said. "It was hard for me. I had a difficult time reading and writing. My thoughts were easily diverted.

"Before I lost my hair I bought two wigs, one long and one short. They were expensive ones and they looked real natural. They were hot and uncomfortable, but I wore them and they looked good. I called them my fantasy hair because I picked styles I hadn't had before.

"My hair came out the first week on chemo. I knew it would. I lost eyebrows, eyelashes—everything. My teenage son and his friends got used to seeing me bald and nobody made a big deal of it. When my hair came back, it was thicker than before, but it also had more gray in it. I'm very grateful for the wisdom of my oncologist in ordering that random biopsy of my other breast. I guess things balance out."

Michelle

Michelle was twenty-eight years old when she felt "a little soreness" in her breast. "I'm religious and I prayed about it and it went away," she said. "But it came back, and when it did, I felt a lump. I decided to go to the doctor because my side also hurt. They did a sonogram and I could see on the screen that it was a big lump."

When the biopsy showed malignancy, Michelle went into shock. "I couldn't believe it. I just kept saying, 'Is this for real?' The doctor said I needed an immediate mastectomy because it was fast growing. I saw an oncologist and a surgeon and they recommended a lumpectomy with radiation and chemotherapy. Everything happened real fast and it wasn't until I got to the hospital that I got scared."

Michelle is separated from her husband and supports her children, who are four, five, six, and ten, with her job as a mail carrier. While she was going through radiation, she was unable to work.

"It took my strength away. I was really tired. My family members kept me going emotionally and so did my religion. The Lord has sheltered me.

"I didn't want a mastectomy, but I would have accepted it if necessary. Instead I just needed the lumpectomy. And I'm fortunate that I had no lymph node involvement. I didn't want to lose my hair, either, and you know what? I didn't! Instead, my hair grew miraculously. I'm a black woman and I had always used chemicals to make it look good. But when I started chemo, my hair went from bad to good. Now it's just as wavy as a baby's. People at my church would say, 'Girl, look at your hair!' I think the Lord touched my hair."

Putting It All Together

Elaine, Beverly, Betsy, and Michelle share a disease and a determination to conquer it. As you are going through treatment, you will meet other breast cancer patients. Observe how they feel about what has happened to them and how that affects their attitude toward themselves, family and friends, their jobs, the medical community, and their futures.

Recovery from breast cancer has an important emotional component. It can work for you or against you. That part of the battle is up to you.

14 Why You: Were You Singled Out to Get Breast Cancer?

It's natural to feel that you've somehow been singled out when you discover that you have breast cancer. "Why me?" may be the first words out of your mouth. The shock and the bitterness may last for weeks—only to develop into depression. And no matter how else you're feeling, you're likely to feel fear and helplessness.

In spite of the advances in treatment, cancer—any kind of cancer—is still equated in many people's minds with an inevitable and painful death. Though the treatment of cancer, and especially breast cancer, has come a long, long way, the prognosis can still be uncertain when it has metastasized. Because you must now put your well-being in the hands of doctors, most or all of whom will be unknown to you, it's normal that you be frightened.

Anger is also a normal response.

"I was angry and I was frightened and I kept wondering 'Why me?'" said Elaine. "I didn't smoke, I ate the right foods, I took care of myself. I was very angry at God. But then I realized that illness is not from God. And then I said, 'Why *not* me?' Somehow, I vowed, I would use this experience for good. I had always known that life was precious, and I'd never been materialistic. But I used the time while I was sick to get to know myself better. As difficult as the whole experience was, some good did come from it."

Elaine's accepting attitude helped her to cope. She tried to make the best of every situation and to help people around her feel better. And she came out a winner.

Betsy also found herself asking "Why me?" But, she said, "I didn't say it as much as other people do. I've studied terminal illness. I've seen too much. I know the roller coaster of emotions cancer patients experience. I tried to stay cool and clinical about everything, and that drove the doctors nuts. They would ask my husband if I knew just how seriously ill I was. I knew precisely, but I refused to break down in front of the doctors. In private I would do that. But I felt that doctors need patients who are in control. This is a tough disease, and I had to fight it in my own way."

You Didn't Wish This Upon Yourself

No one is singled out to get cancer. It just happens. Some people are at higher risk than others—but often the people at highest risk never get it. Cancer is not a punishment, nor do we wish it upon ourselves.

Several books have appeared lately that have suggested that people who get cancer or can't recover from it somehow wish it upon themselves. *This is ridiculous!* It's criminal to suggest that you can cure yourself of your breast cancer. Do not, for a moment, entertain this notion. You will help yourself if you have a courageous attitude and if you will fully cooperate with your prescribed treatment. *But you still need the treatment!*

Western medicine—the type practiced in the United States—still holds the most promise for containment and cure. While you will want to be an active partner in your treatment team, you can rest assured that we currently know more about breast cancer and how to treat it than we ever did before.

Getting Your Stress Under Control

Most cancer patients feel they are under stress. Getting in control of it depends on what works for you. If you've never been to a cancer support group, you may find this very helpful. Talking to other women who've been through the breast cancer experience may prove to be a valuable outlet for your pent-up emotions. If the medical center where you're receiving treatment has no such group, think about starting one. Medical personnel can help you get in touch with other patients and with former patients who would be interested in such a group.

Perhaps you would prefer to visit with only one or two other women who have had breast cancer. Again, medical personnel can be of help in providing names.

If you have a religious affiliation, your minister, priest, or rabbi may be of special help to you at this time. You may also want to investigate biofeedback as a technique to help you control your stress, or imagery as a way to utilize your inner resources.

Reading everything possible about breast cancer is another method that may help you feel more in control. That's what Beverly did.

"When I started out, I knew very little and I read everything I could find," she said. "Some of it scared me, but that was better than not knowing. I felt much more in control once I understood the disease and what was happening to me."

You know yourself best. Try what you think is right for you. And if one thing doesn't work, go on to the next one. Emotional recovery is very much a part of your battle against breast cancer.

The Year Following Surgery

Women who are older, married longer, and perceive that they have support from their families and their doctors reportedly do better during the first year after surgery than their counterparts.

But almost all women report symptoms of distress after having surgery, and it usually doesn't peak until two or three months afterward. This is understandable. It's hard to feel okay about things when physically you feel worse than you did at the time of diagnosis. And it's hard to think about the future when you're fearful the cancer might return or that you'll never be able to pay off all your medical bills.

Consider Professional Help

If your anxiety or depression is incapacitating, you may want to think about some counseling. For this to be successful, it is important that, if at all possible, you see a counselor who works with cancer patients. It may be that the hospital or medical center where you are receiving treatment has a social worker who can assist you, or a psychologist on staff who will help you.

Professional assistance may seem costly, but if you are seeing a skilled counselor, you will consider it well worth the price.

Seek Out Survivors

As depressing as it can be to go for treatment and to be surrounded by other cancer patients, many of whom may seem hopeless and passive, it's important that, whenever you can, you surround yourself with people who make you feel good. These may be family members, friends, or people who have successfully overcome cancer.

Several fine books about overcoming cancer have been published. Finding and reading these may also be helpful to you. A number of them are discussed in the Recommended Resources section at the end of this book.

Your Individualized Approach

As with so many things in life, what you must do is *find what works for you.* If it's a freshly baked croissant and a steaming cup of cappuccino to get you out of bed in the morning, and two video movies before you go to sleep at night, indulge yourself and do whatever it takes to get you through this stressful time.

15 Going Back to Work

Each woman reacts to misfortune in her own way. You may be a person who easily and graciously accepts the sympathy offered by others, or you may be a very private person who cringes at having anyone know your personal business.

Friends and family love you. While coworkers care about you, their major concern may be whether your illness will inconvenience them.

Most of your coworkers will react with sympathy when they hear you have breast cancer. It's difficult—if not impossible—to find a family who isn't touched by cancer in one way or another. At the very least, everyone knows what cancer is (as opposed to some rare disease few people have heard of).

But sympathy can quickly turn into indifference, resentment, and even hostility. Trying to deal with these feelings is especially difficult at a time when you need as much emotional support as possible.

Typical Scenarios

Unfortunately, you may work with the type of person who has the mistaken notion that one wishes a major illness upon oneself, or that one somehow deserves it. Consequently, once past the initial relief that it's you instead of her who is sick, such a coworker may actually act hostile and uncaring toward you. If you allow it, such a person can make you feel even worse than you already do. It's going to be up to you to put this type of reaction in perspective so that it bothers you as little as possible. You need your emotional energy for more important things.

Then there are the coworkers who will say, "Hi, welcome back. You look great!" and then never say another word. Essentially they're telling you, "Okay, that's over. Now get back to work and we'll pretend this never happened."

At the very least you're recovering from major surgery, and if you're trying to work while going through radiation and/or chemotherapy, everything most certainly is *not* back to normal—even if you *do* look great.

Others may gaze at you with anxious looks on their faces—and avoid you whenever possible. You'll wonder if they think what you have is catching, or if your mere presence is a reminder to them that they, too, are mortal and may have to deal sometime with a life-threatening illness.

And there's always the person who will assume that

now that you've had a significant medical experience, you'll want to hear all about every operation *they've* had, as well as those of every immediate relative and their friends and neighbors. You may find yourself wondering how so many obnoxious, overbearing people could ever be employed in the same workplace.

Find the People Who Are Helpful

Fortunately, in most work settings you're also going to find coworkers who are sympathetic and caring and who will be there to help in any way they can. This is the type of person who will offer to drive you to and from work to help you conserve energy and who will cover for you when you need to rest or go to treatment. This is also the person who will cheer you up when you get down and who will listen to your concerns.

"I knew from a psychological perspective that I was better off working," commented Betsy. "I work with wonderful people and they picked up the slack for me when I couldn't travel or when I was so tired I couldn't get a project finished when I said I would. My colleagues created a big support system around me and I knew I could ask them for any kind of help."

Betsy was also very honest with her coworkers about her situation and how she felt about it. Because she felt comfortable, coworkers were able to feel comfortable, too.

Beverly was fortunate to have a business partner who took over the lion's share of the work during the year she was on chemotherapy "and operating at 40 percent. I got my chemo on Wednesday mornings, went home to rest for an hour, and then went back to the office. I made myself work, and I think that was good for me. It helped me to not dwell on my worries. I had other things to think about.

"It was a difficult time for me. Lots of days I didn't feel like working, but I did as much as I could," she recalled. "There are only nine of us in the agency and everyone was very supportive."

When Michelle found she could not work while she was undergoing radiation and had to take a disability leave without pay after her sick leave and vacation time were used up, her coworkers at the post office took up a fund for her, collecting over five hundred dollars to help her pay her bills.

"It was near Christmas and they brought over toys for the kids, so they had a good Christmas, and they brought us food and things like toothpaste and paper towels. People on my mail route gave us food and money.

"When I got sick, I found out what great people I work with," Michelle said with a smile. "I'll never forget their kindness."

One woman we know reported that returning to work proved to be extremely stressful for her. "Our company was having some financial problems and had cut back on staff," she related. "Everyone was having to work overtime and morale was low. Right in the middle of all this I had to be gone for surgery. Then, after I returned to work, I missed two hours every day for five weeks in order to go for my radiation treatment—and then for the next six months I missed a half day every week for my chemo treatments. On top of it, I didn't have much energy and I was pretty emotional and would cry easily."

This woman got mixed signals from her boss. "She seemed sympathetic, yet she also seemed angry when I couldn't keep up with my work. At one point she suggested that I was taking off more time than I really needed to. I got really upset about that and mentioned it to my oncologist. My oncologist called my boss and talked to her. In one way it helped because my boss didn't hassle me anymore. But she acted more aloof after that and I felt like I was treated like the office albatross everyone simply had to tolerate. The whole reaction around the office made me hate my job. I would have quit, but I had to have the income and my health insurance. I knew I'd never get another job if a prospective employer knew I had cancer."

Discrimination Against People Who Have Had Cancer

This woman was correct in assuming that had she quit, she might have had difficulty finding another job. She was able to stay with her job, and fortunately, things gradually got better. But some people can't do their work and do quit. When they want to go back to work, pickings can be slim. Many employers fear that people who have had cancer are a poor insurance risk or may miss too many workdays.

You should be aware that if you apply for a job with a company or business that receives any type of federal funding, you may be able to file a discrimination complaint if you believe you were turned down solely because you have had cancer. The government's Rehabilitation Act is designed to protect the handicapped, and it includes cancer as a handicap. While you may not appreciate that classification, the law can come to your aid. In addition, some states have laws prohibiting discrimination against cancer patients.

Plan Your Return to Work Ahead of Time

You may be able to avoid some problems you might otherwise encounter if you plan your return to work ahead of time. This doesn't mean you can foresee—and prevent—every difficulty you may encounter, because some will be unforeseen. But foresight *can* make things go more smoothly.

Consider what type of job you have and what kind of treatment you will be going through when deciding whether and how much you should work during the first year after surgery.

Begin by asking your oncologist to tell you as realistically as possible if you can work full-time.

If you will be undergoing normal-intensity chemotherapy for six to twelve months, are otherwise in good health, have a supportive husband and/or a network of friends and no small children to care for, and if you have a low-stress office job where you can afford to miss a few hours or a day of work every now and then, chances are you can continue to work full-time—provided you don't suffer adverse side effects, such as chronic nausea and fatigue.

But if you must stand on your feet all day and are getting aggressive chemotherapy that will drastically lower your white blood count, you may have to take a leave of absence or drop back to part-time work. In some businesses, every effort will be made to place you in a desk job temporarily so you can continue to work—but not all employers can be, or are willing to be, that flexible.

If you work in a job where you come in contact with ill people or with small children, you may need to wear a mask to protect yourself from illness or quit work for a while.

Don't Wait for Disaster to Happen

Very few women breeze through radiation and/or chemotherapy without side effects. At the very least, you are likely to suffer tiredness. At most, you may suffer nausea, headaches, hair loss, fatigue, and because of the hormonal changes your body is going through, unpredictable mood swings.

Some women going through chemotherapy or hormone therapy experience an almost instant menopause. This is not the way Mother Nature intended it to be, and you may find yourself mired in depression or experiencing fits of anger and frustration that you can't explain and can't control. If you are also trying to deal with an uncooperative boss, hostile coworkers, and too much to do, you may feel like you're ready to explode.

One way to ease through this is to have an alternative arrangement agreed to ahead of time with your employer. You may need to be switched to a different work task or take several weeks off, or your employer may need to hire a temporary worker if you're going to be going through intense chemotherapy. If your employer knows this ahead of time, everything will go more smoothly when the time comes.

Perhaps you can arrange with a coworker to do a time-share: If that person will take on extra work for you now, you'll pay him or her back once you're better by assuming their extra work for the same amount of time.

Again, the secret of success is making sure that everybody knows about the arrangement ahead of time and has agreed to it so there are no unpleasant surprises and people don't get angry with you.

The Plight of the Working Mother

Working women with young children who are either single parents or have hostile or uncooperative spouses have the worst time getting through the treatment phase. Even before their illness they had no wiggle room in their lives. When they fall ill, they are often more worried about the repercussions on their families than about their own health.

Too many of them continue to try to do it all—and end up collapsing from exhaustion.

Remember: *Surgery is not the end of your battle against cancer—it's just the beginning!*

If you are that mother of young children who is also trying to hold down a job, try to remember what it was like when you were pregnant. Chances are, you directed all of your energies toward the welfare of your unborn child. You would have done whatever it took to have a successful pregnancy and birth. You would have done anything for your baby, including going into debt if extra medical care had been needed.

Now you've got to think the same way about your own life. The bottom line is, do you want to leave your children without a mother? Of course not! So you must take good care of yourself. You must do whatever it takes to get yourself healthy again. If that means a few months off work, then that's what you should do. If it means dropping that MBA program or dropping some clubs and organizations, do it. *Take care of you!*

That must be your job now. That is where you must direct your energies. Ask your spouse or lover, friends, and relatives to help you with the children and with housework. Arrange for someone else to take that business trip for you. Have a heart-to-heart talk with your employer so you can arrange for extra time. Perhaps you won't need it—but at least it will then be there if you do.

How you treat yourself during the first year after your cancer diagnosis will influence your health for years to come. Find the people who are willing to help you out. And remember that any sacrifice you make for your health is worth it.

<u>16</u> Friends and Family

One of the hard issues you must deal with in the course of your illness is its impact upon family and friends.

To some degree, the way they will react will depend upon you. But in spite of your best intentions, some of them will disappoint you.

Friendship on the Line

Cancer is a scary word, and when your friends hear about you, their responses will vary. All of them will be very sorry for you. But like the people you work with if you have a job, some will find themselves incapable of reaching out to you. Either they don't know what to say, are afraid of saying the wrong thing, or they don't want to have to think about what you're going through—because it's a painful reminder that it could happen to them or to a loved one.

"Close friends kept me going," commented Elaine. "I have several who have just been great. I'm so thankful for them. But," she said, "being around a group of people I considered friends was different. The word 'cancer' has an enormous stigma attached to it. It silences a room. People are afraid they'll say something wrong. So what I did was to talk about it and make people comfortable with it."

"I had one girlfriend I could call up and we'd cry together," remembered Michelle. "I'm what you'd call a loner, but people I didn't even know were my friends helped me through this. I found the more support you get from others, the better you feel."

And while most women find that at least a few friends will stick right with them and help them in any way possible, others they would have expected to be there for them faded away.

It may be hard to believe, but some people still think cancer is contagious. That being near someone who has it, or even thinking about it, can cause it. If you suspect a friend of believing this, or of not being in touch because he or she simply doesn't know what to say to you, it may be up to you to make the first contact and try to put that person at ease.

What you may find out is that your friend was waiting for a signal from you to find out what he or she could do for you. Your friend might have thought you didn't want company or that you'd know you could ask for help if you needed it. This type of friend needs direction from you and, once the ice has been broken, will be there for you.

You may think that you have enough to occupy your thoughts without having to reach out to friends as well. After all, isn't it their job to reach out to you? But you will probably find that reaching out to others makes you feel good and is well worth the effort.

At the other extreme may be the friend who wants to take over your life for you. Such "do-gooders" can be a real problem. You may be very glad to have help, but it's also important that you stay in control of your life and that one or two people don't become overly intrusive in your personal life. Let your friend know you are grateful for assistance, but don't relinquish control.

Most friends will fall somewhere in the middle. They want to do something to help, whether you need an errand run or just want some company. Believe people when they say, "If there's anything I can do for you, just call me." Chances are, they really mean it.

If you are new in the place where you live or if you don't have many friends, this may be an especially lonely time for you. If you will reach out, you will find new friends. By informing your physician, a visiting nurse, or a member of the clergy that you are lonely and would appreciate some company, you will be put in touch with other cancer patients or with volunteers who will be glad to pass some time with you. But it is up to you to make your needs known.

Michelle found that members of her church not only befriended her, but also offered practical assistance.

"They brought us food and came in and cared for the children and even washed and ironed our clothes," she said. "My church became my support system. I hope I can help someone else the way those people helped me."

Going through an experience like cancer will probably teach you very quickly who your real friends are. They will stay close to you and do whatever they can for you. There will be others you may never hear from again. Having to accept that can be heartbreaking. Most cancer patients will tell you they had the same thing happen to them.

How Children React to Mom's Cancer

If you have children, you have yet another concern, because your illness affects your children—even if it doesn't seem to.

Your family is also experiencing your illness. Medical personnel and friends may view them as bystanders, but they are very much involved in what is happening to you, even if one or more family members seem indifferent or uncaring.

Your role in the family will be different for a while, and adjusting to that is a task for them as well as you. Families need support, too. They feel shock, anger, helplessness, and depression.

That feeling of helplessness is especially difficult to deal with. And they feel more helpless if they aren't able to talk openly about their fears and to communicate directly to medical personnel. They *need* to participate in the treatment plan so they can feel they are contributing something positive to what is otherwise a negative, scary situation.

Because of the disruption caused by your illness, members of your family may feel blame, guilt, shame, and ambivalence. In families where there is a lot of conflict in the best of times, these feelings may be almost overwhelming when a crisis like breast cancer comes along.

In spite of all the attention that must be paid to your illness, children need to continue to go to school and to lead normal lives. But at the same time, they have a need to offer you special care and attention.

Often families must realign their roles so that your tasks are absorbed in the event that you can't do them. While this can create conflict, it is also a good opportunity for family members to feel they are doing something important and something that helps you.

Long-Term Impact on Children

One of your fears may be that your children will be permanently scarred by the trauma of witnessing a life-threatening illness. But long-term studies show that children have a natural resiliency in the face of such difficulties, and if you help them, most of them will adapt well and will be without long-term consequences.

How your children perceive your illness will depend in large part on their ages. In a study of children ages seven to sixteen, researchers drew the following conclusions:

Children seven to ten worry about the family unit and about what will happen next. They commonly say they feel scared, lonely, worried, and sometimes angry. They wonder how their mothers got sick. They need to know that they will be cared for and that the family will remain intact.

Children who are ten to thirteen are preoccupied with their own role and will comment on what the disruption at home means to them. For example, they may have to help around the house more or are expected to behave more maturely. They need more specific information than younger children about treatment and prognosis. They need their self-sufficiency supported.

Adolescents are typically in the process of withdrawing from the closeness they've formerly shared with their parents, so a crisis like breast cancer is a real test for them. They want to be more independent just at the time their families need them most. Most adolescents will experience guilt and conflict.

Most mothers say that going through an illness like breast cancer is much tougher when there are children in the home. Young children, of course, still need much physical care, but don't necessarily understand the gravity of the situation. Older children worry about their mothers, but may be afraid to show it.

Include Your Children in What's Happening

Children of all ages may feel better if they are allowed to visit the cancer treatment center so they can view the equipment and meet the people who help you. If that's not possible, it's important that you or someone else explain to them just what happens to you when you go for treatment and why you may not feel well afterward.

Don't assume children are too young to understand. They need this information, and if it's explained simply and clearly, they'll understand what they need to satisfy them.

Michelle involved her daughters, ages four, five, and six, in the care of her catheter. Her daughters would take turns bringing her the cleaning solutions and watch while she did the cleaning. This allowed them to feel they had participated in her care. "I let them be part of it so they wouldn't be afraid of it," Michelle said.

Her ten-year-old son had to take over more work at home. Michelle tried to keep it simple for him. He would prepare TV dinners for everyone and help get his sisters ready for bed.

Communication Is Important

Adjustments, such as who's going to clean house and do the grocery shopping, can be difficult in a family. Families who have always been good about sharing feelings and about working together will have a much easier time with all this than families who have communication problems.

A support group for cancer patients and their families, such as "I Can Cope" or "Make Today Count," can be a place where family members can discuss their feelings and receive support and feedback from other group members. It may also be wise to talk individually and together with a social worker skilled in working with the families of cancer patients in order to give each family member necessary support and reinforcement.

Talking with Children About Cancer

It's important that you not give children too great a burden to bear regarding your illness or you may cause them such emotional distress that their normal functioning and development are impaired.

Encourage children to ask what's on their minds and answer their questions honestly. If you feel too emotional to do this, your spouse, lover, a relative, friend, or your doctor may be willing to do it. Relatives and friends can also assist by spending extra time with your children if they are young so they don't feel neglected and to give them the guidance and affection they need.

Michelle found that her son was reluctant to discuss her illness. After questioning him, she learned that he thought cancer was caused by smoking.

"I had always told him that your body is a temple and you shouldn't abuse it with drugs, alcohol, or smoking. So he was afraid I had been smoking in secret and cancer was my punishment. He was very relieved when I reassured him that I hadn't smoked."

Together, Michelle and her children watched a Peanuts' Charlie Brown special on children and cancer. While the program was about children who have cancer, it provided the opening to discuss all sorts of things, such as the fact that her hair might fall out when she was taking radiation and chemotherapy.

"I'm really thankful for that show," she said. "It let us talk."

Beverly found her adult son and daughter to be "very sympathetic. They tried to cheer me up. Both of them were sensitive to my feelings and my condition and I talked with them regularly."

Betsy was very open and honest with her sons, who were twenty-three and sixteen, but "weren't really involved in all this." Neither was at home at the time her cancer was diagnosed and she went in for surgery, so they missed one of the critical times.

Because Elaine has two daughters, ages twenty and twenty-three, she worried about their reaction, knowing they are now at higher risk for getting the disease themselves. "Both of my daughters have been very concerned for me," she said. "My daughter in New York flew home four times the first year. My other daughter lives at home and has been quite upset. We had a psychologist talk briefly to them. This has to be hard for them."

The Risk to Adult Daughters

Indeed, the risk to daughters of breast cancer mothers is higher than it is for the normal population—but this varies tremendously, depending on the age of the mother at diagnosis, whether one or both breasts were involved, and whether other family members have also had breast cancer. The risk can be as little as 11 percent or as high as 35 percent, depending on some of these factors.

Sisters of these women also face an increased risk, but mothers may feel guilty for the danger they're passing on to their daughters, while daughters may feel anger toward their mothers. This is an emotionally charged issue that bears more study than it's been given thus far by social scientists.

Getting Through This Together

There was a time not long ago when cancer patients were often not told what was wrong with them. Although most of them guessed the truth, the conspiracy to keep the sick person from knowing his or her own diagnosis created an artificial atmosphere in which the illness could not be discussed.

Today we know that cancer patients and their loved ones are much better off if they can discuss what is happening and reveal their feelings honestly.

Adjustment can take time. Each family member has to deal with his or her own feelings. While you are the one who is sick and the one with the most at stake, it's important that you let family members express how they're feeling and willingly listen to them, even if they feel anger toward you because of the impact your illness is having on *their* lives. (Just remember that they are actually angry with the illness and not with you.)

If you can openly and honestly communicate with each other, you will be able to weather this bad time and fully enjoy the good times that are sure to be part of your future.

17 Living with and Loving the New You

When you're diagnosed with breast cancer, your foremost concern is making the right decisions regarding your health. With surgery behind you and your attention focused on your life ahead, one issue you may wrestle with is overcoming your bitterness that you have gotten cancer. Another is coming to terms with your own sexuality.

Women who have had mastectomies may have the most difficult time with this. In spite of your husband or lover's reassurances to the contrary, you may wonder how any man could ever find you desirable again.

Learning to accept and love yourself as you now are and reestablishing your identity as a sexual being may take some time. Undergoing breast reconstruction may or may not help.

A mastectomy is a violation of the body—an amputation of a body part. Your breast was an integral part of your image as a woman. And even if you undergo reconstruction, you may never feel like that new "breast" is really you.

Some women battle a long time with feelings of inadequacy—a sense that they are no longer a real woman. They can argue with themselves that it was "just a breast, a useless appendage, something I can live without," yet they can't come to terms with the loss.

In her book *The Cancer Journals*, feminist writer Audre Lorde recounts her experience of going through a mastectomy and her recovery. When she finally accepts that her breast is gone, she speaks of the grief she felt: "My right breast represented such an area of feeling and pleasure for me, how could I bear never to feel that again?"

As she struggles to "love my body one-breasted now, or remain forever alien to myself," she reexamines her life and the values she lives by, concluding that she is still whole inside and that now that she is free of the cancer that threatened her survival, life can still be very rewarding.

Your Grief Is Real

To grieve for the missing breast is natural and should be recognized as such. Any kind of grief must be allowed to run its course if emotional healing is to take place.

You shouldn't apologize for the way you're feeling, nor should you let anyone make you feel guilty for grieving for your lost breast. Others may try to tell you that you should be grateful that your life has been spared. "Look at the women who have advanced cancer," they will say.

And of course you know that, and you *are* grateful. But your grief is still real and profound and your healing must be emotional and psychological and spiritual as well as physical.

How you feel about yourself as time proceeds is very important. Some women become mired in depression and it can take years for them to recover their former self-esteem and learn to accept their altered bodies. In the meantime, their feelings can negatively impact other important areas of life.

Reaching a State of Acceptance

That your self-concept has been altered and your self-esteem battered cannot be argued. After the anger and rage subside, after grieving runs its course, you must reach a degree of acceptance and learn how to get on with life.

What Does "Sexy" Mean?

Unfortunately we live in a society that emphasizes the female breast and its role in a woman's sexual attractiveness. Because of this, many women assume their spouses or lovers—or future spouses or lovers—cannot possibly find them sexy and desirable. Sometimes this becomes a self-fulfilling prophecy if the woman reacts by assuming she's undesirable and acts accordingly.

Feeling that her desirability is based on her breasts

is buying into an attitude that is unfair to most men. Several studies show that when women have mastectomies, regardless of whether they lose one or both breasts, only a very few husbands consider them less desirable sexually.

Husbands Worry Most About Wives' Health

Husbands' greatest concerns are invariably centered on their wives' health. Loss of breasts is insignificant in comparison. Sexuality is not body parts, and most men know this very well.

Sexuality is everything you are, from your sense of humor to your intellect to the way you conduct yourself in everyday activities. It's how you make your partner feel emotionally in bed, as opposed to what a body part feels like. If you can accept yourself as you now are— whether or not you have reconstruction—that will make all the difference in terms of your sex appeal.

Reestablishing Your Sex Life After Surgery

This is not to say that reestablishing a sexual relationship may not be difficult. But the reason is not your lost breast or breasts. It's because too many couples don't know how to communicate about sexual matters.

You may find that your husband has seemingly lost interest in sex and you may feel rejected. "I'm not sexy anymore. I only have one breast. He's probably already having an affair—and who could blame him? Look at me. I'm not complete. I'm going to lose my husband because of this."

And while you torture yourself with this scenario, the truth of the matter may be that your husband has not initiated sex because he's feeling overprotective of you. He's afraid of hurting you—or he's afraid that given what you've been through, *you're* not interested in sex and he's waiting for some sort of signal from you.

Diminished Sex Drive Is also a Possibility

It's also possible that you don't have the sexual drive you had before. Your husband is interested in sex and you aren't. Poor body image may be only part of your problem. Depending on the kind of surgery you had, and your follow-up treatment, your body may be going through many hormonal changes. You may be in the middle of a crash menopause, suffering from hot flashes.

Sudden menopause is not the way Mother Nature intended it to be and it can cause tremendous emotional upheaval. Intercourse may be uncomfortable because your vagina is dry. You may be under a lot of stress and suffering from depression. *How in the world can you expect to feel sexy!*

Recognize the Problem and Find a Solution

Open, honest communication is the key to solving all or any of these problems. You must share your feelings and your concerns. Your doctor can prescribe an antidepressant to help you cope with depression and mood swings. There are medicines, lubricants, and vaginal creams to moisten and/or thicken the vaginal lining so that intercourse is once again comfortable.

Your doctor can also assist you by visiting with your

husband and explaining medically what you are going through. A counselor or therapist may also be of assistance if the two of you can't explore your feelings about your illness and its impact on your relationship. Working with you individually and together, a good therapist can help you recognize and vent pent-up feelings and get you back on track.

In the beginning it may be necessary to refrain from sex and to be content with holding and cuddling each other. Sex will follow naturally if you don't rush the process.

When the Relationship Falls Apart

While this is what often happens in relationships when a woman has a mastectomy, there is, unfortunately, another scenario. While most men will be supportive and loving toward the women they love, a few simply can't offer any emotional support and some of them might even disappear from your life when your cancer is diagnosed.

At a time when you need more support than you've ever needed in your life, you may find your husband or lover denying that anything life threatening is even going on. He may seem impatient with you and expect you to quickly step back into the role you fulfilled before, whether as wife, mother, housekeeper, or paycheck earner.

Chances are, the two of you had communication problems prior to your illness. Several studies have concluded that the key to whether a spouse is supportive after his wife's mastectomy is the degree of their marital satisfaction *before* the mastectomy.

While most couples survive this experience with

their marriage intact and as strong or stronger than before, some marriages are unable to survive this major blow. Chances are, they were coming apart anyway.

Breast cancer can be the catalyst that either jolts the partners into a renewed sense of closeness and commitment or drives them apart. It can exacerbate problems already present in the marriage. It can show partners the other's true nature.

Some couples will remain together for a while because of guilt, or stay together long enough for the woman to regain her health before they part. But from the moment breast cancer is diagnosed, the marriage itself—or the relationship—may be essentially over.

Introducing Your "Infirmity" to a New Sex Partner

Women who are single and who were sexually active before their mastectomies have a different problem. How do you tell a man in whom you are interested that you've had a mastectomy—and what impact does this have on a potential sexual relationship?

This was the dilemma faced by a woman we'll call Erica. She was seriously involved with Darrel when her breast cancer was diagnosed and she had a unilateral mastectomy. Darrel seemed to be in a daze about it all. While he came to the hospital to see her, he acted remote and uncommunicative. When Erica suggested he see her scar, he refused. Once she was out of the hospital and back at work, he left.

Devastated by what she perceived as his rejection, she quickly started a relationship with Tony, a man she was acquainted with at work. Tony knew about her mastectomy and almost from the beginning was *asking* to see the scar. Trying to forget Darrel, Erica started a sexual relationship with Tony, but was quickly put off by what seemed like his morbid interest in her missing breast. She quit seeing him, and for a long time remained celibate.

"And then I met Ron," she recalled. "I knew immediately that this was a man I could be interested in spending the rest of my life with. But how in the world could I tell him that even though I had gone through reconstruction, one breast wasn't the real me?"

Feeling she had to broach the subject *before* they slept together, she told him, very casually, when they were at dinner on their third date, that two years earlier she had been diagnosed with breast cancer and had undergone a mastectomy and reconstruction.

To her immense relief, his concern was only about her health. "When we finally slept together, it was lovely," Erica related. "We're going to be married early next year."

It's only fair that a man you become involved with know of your condition before he finds it out for himself. But, once again, if you are comfortable with it, then you can present it to him the same way, and chances are it will never be an issue of importance to him.

Michelle is presently separated from her husband. He was unable to offer any emotional support to her while she was going through her ordeal, though he did remain actively involved with the children.

"Men back away from things like this," Michelle philosophized. "They say, 'I can't talk to you when you cry.' I guess I didn't expect it to be any different."

Elaine, on the other hand, found her husband to be her chief support system. "He told me I was going to fight this. He's artistic and he was always making these little drawings for me showing things like little men with swords going after my cancer cells. I know this whole ordeal was very hard on him, but he really did support me. He's my partner in the most beautiful way and I know I couldn't get that kind of support from anyone else."

Betsy and Beverly also had supportive spouses. "My husband was the only person I would break down in front of. He was my source of support," Betsy said.

Beverly reported that her husband has been "wonderful. It would have been devastating going through this without him. I think we're closer now than we've ever been before."

I'm Okay, You're Okay

Just remember that above all, men worry about their wives' or lovers' health. Then they worry about how these women they love will react to their illness and to losing a breast. What it will be like making love to a woman with a missing breast or breasts or with reconstructed breasts is minor in comparison.

While you can't always predict how your lover or spouse will react to the reality of your breast cancer, you can be certain that many people—and very likely your spouse or lover—will be looking for cues from you as to how to act. If you practice the "I'm okay, you're okay" school of thought, if your outlook is positive and you're determined to make the best of your ill fortune, those around you—family, friends, and coworkers—will probably act likewise.

The sooner you can accept your new body, whether it's the minor scarring but possible radiation redness of lumpectomy, or a double mastectomy without reconstruction, the sooner others around you can also accept it.

You May Have to Pretend for a While

For a while you may have to fake it. If you go through radiation and/or chemotherapy, you may feel lousy. Your hair may fall out. You hurt. Your body is in hormonal crisis. You have financial problems, you're tired all the time, your children are acting up, and there seems to be no relief in sight. On top of it all, you may be scared to death that your cancer will come back.

This is when you're going to find out what you're really made of. It's a time to affirm the fact that you're alive and that you can still have a wonderful life. You *can* get the problems under control and life *can* be good again.

It will take some work. At a time when you're not feeling good about yourself, you'll need to push yourself to make certain you always look nice when you're with other people. It'll take a lot of courage to tell others about what's happened to you and to endure their questions and perhaps some self-conscious stares. It will be a challenge to communicate your needs to your husband or lover, and to feel comfortable with your changed body.

As we've already suggested, you'll need to find what helps you. It may be meditation or daily prayer. Even repeating an affirmation such as "better better better" as you walk briskly through the park as part of a physical fitness program may be helpful.

18 Be Good to Yourself

During the year following your cancer diagnosis, if you're like most women, you will suffer emotionally and physically. You may feel your world is falling apart. You may wonder if you even want to go on living. You may question God's cruelty to you, wondering why you've been singled out to have breast cancer.

You may go through tremendous hormonal changes, lose your hair, lose or gain weight, and may have to go through the difficult adjustment to disfiguring surgery. You may face the prospect of more surgery—and feel scared to death about it.

You may dread the future, not knowing what your prognosis is. You may blame and praise your doctors all in one breath. And you may think nobody understands what you're going through—except other women going through it or who have gone through it.

Cancer patients must live with a great deal of stress. Given all the attention devoted to the topic of stress these days, you know the toll it can take on you physically and mentally. We've already discussed the need to get it under control in your life and ways to do it.

Part of getting stress under control is accepting the bitterness you feel about what has happened to you— and then letting it go. Bitterness can eat at you and destroy you. But as we all learn sooner or later in life, bad things happen to good people. You didn't deserve cancer. It just happened. Medical science is searching hard for prevention and cure, but it has a long way to go. Doctors say the wrong things to patients, friends say the wrong things, spouses and children say the wrong things. Depression sweeps over you like a wave. Medical bills pile up and you have no energy.

But you know already that life's like that. This may be the hardest year in your life, but it's only a year.

How you get through it—defeated by bitterness or in control of your life—is up to you.

Some people keep up their spirits by helping others. Getting your mind off yourself and your troubles can be very effective therapy. Others release stress and make themselves feel better by starting a physical fitness program that gets them out of the house and around nature and other people. Find what meets your needs. Find what's right for you.

You must love yourself. Make peace with your new physical self—and know that whatever you look like on the outside, what truly counts is what's on the inside. And that the people in this life who truly count will think so, too.

If you can do these things, there will be a tremendous payback. Though, as a result of your ordeal, you may have lost some friends, you will have made others. You will have learned to know yourself, and you will have learned how very precious life is—something few people ever recognize. And knowing that, how can anything outside yourself ever have control over you again?

A FINAL WORD

Hope. That's the final word. Even as you read this, research is going on all over the world into the causes and treatments for cancer. Breast cancer receives a great deal of attention because it affects such huge numbers of women.

Technology races forward. And as we learn more, survival rates for women with breast cancer get better and better. Surgery and treatment become more exacting. The suffering of patients is lessened.

Right now there are many promising research programs under way. Cancer researchers are developing better anticancer drugs with fewer side effects, antinausea medications, and improved radiation therapy. They're seeking ways to make surgery less mutilating and to protect the rest of body from damage during follow-up treatment, even very intense chemotherapy.

They're also searching for ways to prevent cancer and to predict who is at risk for it so these people can take special precautions.

Research is under way to learn how to sample very small amounts of breast tissue in order to test for abnormal amounts of chromosomal material or abnormal amounts of different proteins or gene products that may predict which women will get breast cancer.

Also in the works is a search for the appropriate preventive measures that may then be instituted in the woman at very high risk for developing breast cancer. These measures may include preventive medications (such as tamoxifen or vitamin-A derivatives) or prophylactic surgery (removing the breasts to prevent the development of breast cancer), and special attention to diet and hormone ingestion. Some foods contain natural cancer preventives. Research is under way to extract these preventive chemicals and add them in large amounts to food we normally eat.

And there is continuous research into hormone replacement therapy for postmenopausal women in order to treat them without placing them at increased risk for breast cancer.

Preventive research is especially exciting. Scientists are seeking the reason women who drink alcohol and smoke are at higher risk for getting breast cancer, and why excess fat in the diet also puts women at increased risk.

The Hereditary Cancer Institute at Creighton University in Omaha, Nebraska, as well as other universities are studying families with a high incidence of cancer, searching for those genes responsible for passing cancer from generation to generation.

Cancer and the Mind

In the realm of the psychological, more and more is being learned about cancer and the mind.

We know without question that cancer patients with a strong will to live and to recover do better than the patients who are less resolved. A strong religious faith, family, and support groups enable patients to handle whatever comes their way more effectively.

While there is still much to learn about the connections between the mind and cancer—and it is a field of intense investigation—we do know that a courageous attitude, a sense of inner peace, and a willingness to follow a prescribed course of medical therapy yields more positive results than any other form of treatment.

Your battle against cancer is one you probably never thought you'd have to undertake. Marshal all your reserves—your faith, your intelligence, your basic health, your spirit and drive—and give this battle everything you've got.

Whatever your prognosis, remember that the key word is "hope." *Never give up.* More women than ever before are living happy, productive lives for many years after their breast cancer was initially diagnosed.

RECOMMENDED RESOURCES

The American Cancer Society: This volunteer organization has chapters throughout the country to assist cancer patients and their families with information, transportation, equipment loan or rental, volunteer visitors, support groups for specific types of cancer, and financial assistance. ACS receives no government subsidies.

"Reach to Recovery" is a program run by trained volunteers who have had breast cancer. They visit with women newly diagnosed with cancer and offer emotional support and practical information.

"I Can Cope" is an eight-session educational program for cancer patients and their families. They receive current information from health professionals and have the opportunity to meet and socialize with other families living with cancer.

Your local chapter of the American Cancer Society will be able to tell you what support groups are in your area and how to get in touch with them. If you do not find a local chapter of the ACS listed in your phone directory, write or call the national office between the hours of eight A.M. and five P.M. weekdays for the name of the chapter nearest you.

American Cancer Society
P.O. Box 22200
Atlanta, GA 30322
(404) 320-3333
Toll free: 1-800-227-2345

Encore (Encouragement, Normalcy, Counseling, Opportunity, Reaching Out, Energies Revived) is a support program sponsored by the National YWCA for postoperative breast cancer patients. Group meetings focus on exercise and discussion. For information on a chapter near you, contact:

YWCA—National Office
126 Broadway
New York, NY 10003

Make Today Count is a self-help organization for people with any type of life-threatening illness. It provides peer support through a buddy system that focuses on improving the quality of one's life, despite chronic illness. For information, contact:

Make Today Count
P.O. Box 22
Osage Beach, MO 65065
(314) 348-1619

The National Cancer Institute: Funded by the U.S. Department of Health and Human Services, the NCI offers free publications about cancer upon request, and has a large selection on a diversity of topics from diet to adjuvant treatment.

The NCI also sponsors a Cancer Information Service staffed by professionals and trained volunteers. They can be reached Monday through Saturday and will process requests for written materials and answer medical and technical questions. Up-to-date information on treatment and listings of cancer specialists in your area is also available. For information on the National Cancer Institute and its services, call 1-800-4-CANCER.

PDQ (Physician Data Query): One especially valuable service offered by the NCI is a computerized information service called PDQ. By calling the NCI at 1-800-4-CANCER, you can receive up-to-date information about physicians and treatment centers in your area, the latest cancer treatment information, and an explanation of clinical trials and ones currently in progress.

The information on breast cancer, for example, describes PDQ and its services, and explains breast cancer and its various treatments in clear, simple language. It also lists publications available through NCI that you may wish to request.

External Reconstruction Technology: For information on custom-designed breast prosthesis, contact External Reconstruction Technology at 4835 Benner St., Philadelphia, PA 19135, (215) 333-5440. They will send you descriptive information and/or put you in touch with the consultant in your area.

Recommended Reading

Beauty and Cancer by Diane Doan Noyes and Peggy Mellody, R.N. Los Angeles: AC Press, 1988, $12.95. Full of valuable tips on hair alternatives, special clothing, makeup techniques, and information on diet, exercise, skin care, insurance reimbursement, and more for women going through cancer treatment. Written by a former cancer patient and an R.N. Easy to understand, well illustrated.

The Cancer Conquerors by Greg Anderson. Kansas City: Andrews & McMeel, 1988, $7.95. A cancer survivor once given thirty days to live, Anderson shares a program of beliefs, choices, life decisions, and spiritual growth to help cancer patients overcome fear and uncertainty. Anderson tells a parable of his own "incredible journey to wellness."

The Cancer Journals by Audre Lorde, Spinsters/Aunt Lute Book Company, 1980, $7.00. In a powerful narrative, poet Audre Lorde relates her personal experience with breast cancer and its impact upon her life and work.

I Can Cope by Judi Johnson, R.N., Ph.D., and Linda Klein. Minneapolis: DCI Publishing, 1988. Subtitled "Staying Healthy with Cancer," this book discusses everything from diagnosis to treatment options, to dealing with side effects and learning new ways to communicate with friends, family, and medical personnel. A readable book full of practical, helpful advice for all cancer patients.

When Bad Things Happen to Good People by Harold S. Kushner. New York: Avon Books, 1981, $3.95. Whether or not you are religious, you may find comfort in Rabbi Kushner's classic treatise on misfortune and the human reaction to it. A short, very readable paperback.

Glossary

ADJUVANT THERAPY—Treatment with chemotherapy or hormone therapy after all known tumor has been removed with surgery and/or radiation.

AREOLA—Circular area of darkened skin that surrounds the nipple.

ASPIRATION—A procedure that employs a hollow needle to withdraw fluid from a breast mass.

BENIGN—Without cancer.

BIOPSY—Removal of tissue to test for cancer.

CANCER—A group of diseases (over one hundred) characterized by out-of-control, abnormal cell growth.

CATHETER—a tube implanted or inserted into the body to inject or withdraw fluid.

CHEMOTHERAPY—Treatment with powerful drugs capable of destroying cancer cells.

CLINICAL TRIALS—Studies to evaluate new cancer treatments.

CYST—A sac that arises within the body that is filled with liquid or semisolid material.

ESTROGEN—A female hormone.

EXTERNAL BEAM RADIATION—Radiation therapy delivered to the body by a machine located outside the body. The radiation is delivered directly to the site of the cancer.

HORMONE THERAPY—Treating cancer by removing or adding hormones.

IMPLANT RADIATION—Delivering radiation directly to the site of the cancer (tumor bed) through very small tubes surgically placed in the body.

INFUSION—Putting fluids into the veins by letting them drip slowly through a tube.

INTRAVENOUS—Referred to as IV. Inserting fluid directly into the vein by injection or infusion.

LUMPECTOMY—Surgery to remove a cancerous lump in the breast, along with a small surrounding rim of normal tissue.

LYMPH NODES—Small, bean-shaped glands containing many white blood cells that fight infection.

LYMPHEDEMA—A condition characterized by the collection of excess fluid in the hand and arm after lymph nodes are removed or blocked.

MALIGNANT—Cancerous.

MAMMOGRAM—An X-ray picture of the breast that reveals its internal structures.

MASTECTOMY—Surgical removal of the breast.

MASTECTOMY, PROPHYLACTIC—Removing one or both breasts of a woman who is at especially high risk for developing breast cancer but who does not yet have the disease.

METASTASIS—The spread of cancer cells from one location to another. The cancer cells in the new location are like those in the original.

ONCOLOGIST—A physician who specializes in the treatment of cancer.

PATHOLOGIST—A physician who specializes in the diagnosis of disease via the study of cells and tissue.

PROGESTERONE—A female hormone.

TUMOR—An abnormal growth of cells or tissue.

INDEX

Italics indicates illustrations